Oral Diagnostics Tools and Techniques

A physicist's approach

Online at: https://doi.org/10.1088/978-0-7503-5316-8

IPEM–IOP Series in Physics and Engineering in Medicine and Biology

About the Series

The series in Physics and Engineering in Medicine and Biology will allow the Institute of Physics and Engineering in Medicine (IPEM) to enhance its mission to 'advance physics and engineering applied to medicine and biology for the public good'.

It is focused on key areas including, but not limited to:

- clinical engineering
- diagnostic radiology
- informatics and computing
- magnetic resonance imaging
- nuclear medicine
- physiological measurement
- radiation protection
- radiotherapy
- rehabilitation engineering
- ultrasound and non-ionising radiation.

A number of IPEM–IOP titles are being published as part of the EUTEMPE Network Series for Medical Physics Experts.

A full list of titles published in this series can be found here: https://iopscience.iop.org/bookListInfo/physics-engineering-medicine-biology-series.

Oral Diagnostics Tools and Techniques

A physicist's approach

Edited by
Ashutosh Kumar Shukla
Department of Physics, Ewing Christian College, Prayagraj, UP, India

IOP Publishing, Bristol, UK

ISBN 978-0-7503-5316-8 (ebook)
ISBN 978-0-7503-5314-4 (print)
ISBN 978-0-7503-5317-5 (myPrint)
ISBN 978-0-7503-5315-1 (mobi)

DOI 10.1088/978-0-7503-5316-8

Version: 20230901

IOP ebooks

British Library Cataloguing-in-Publication Data: A catalogue record for this book is available from the British Library.

Published by IOP Publishing, wholly owned by The Institute of Physics, London

IOP Publishing, No.2 The Distillery, Glassfields, Avon Street, Bristol, BS2 0GR, UK

US Office: IOP Publishing, Inc., 190 North Independence Mall West, Suite 601, Philadelphia, PA 19106, USA

To my parents

Contents

Preface

I am happy to present this edited volume covering different tools and techniques applied in oral diagnosis that lead to effective treatment planning. This book contains seven chapters which highlight the physical principles behind such tools and techniques. This volume covers a broad range of diagnostic modalities from conventional techniques based on x-rays to state-of-the-art techniques based on electrical conductivity measurement, ultrasound, fiber-optic transillumination, computed tomography, and magnetic resonance imaging. Fluorescence-based devices and many other novel modalities for oral diagnosis are also covered. In addition, this volume presents molecular spectroscopy techniques coupled with chemometrics for such applications. The individual chapters have been freely woven by the expert contributors and hence have the flavors of both academia and practice. A brief account of the historical background of the techniques covered in the individual chapters gives the reader an idea of how the current version of each technique has gradually evolved. This content definitely offers an enriched learning experience for novice researchers and practitioners. A specific chapter has been included to illustrate the mechanism of oral biofilm formation, the diseases it causes, and its treatment using antibiotics and nanoparticles.

I sincerely thank T Michael Slaughter, senior commissioning editor, IOP Publishing for giving me an opportunity to present this volume to an audience. I wish to thank Phoebe Hooper, ebooks editorial assistant, IOP Publishing for extending every support during the different publication stages of this project. I sincerely thank the expert contributors for contributing to this volume in a timely manner and helping me to meet the schedule.

Ashutosh Kumar Shukla
Prayagraj, India
March 2023

Editor biography

Ashutosh Kumar Shukla

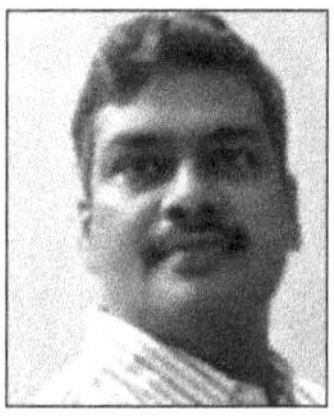

Ashutosh Kumar Shukla has more than two decades of physics teaching and research experience. He has had numerous articles and review articles published in peer-reviewed journals. He has also authored textbooks and participated as an editor in more than 20 edited volumes published by reputed publishers, often prepared in collaboration with experts from different countries. He intends to continue pursuing his academic interests, which include spectroscopic applications in different fields of societal importance.

List of contributors

Guilherme dos Santos Gomes Alves
Postgraduate Program in Health Sciences, University of Western São Paulo (UNOESTE), 19050-920 Presidente Prudente/São Paulo, Brazil

Wilmer Ramirez Carmona
Department of Preventive and Restorative Dentistry, School of Dentistry, Araçatuba, São Paulo State University (Unesp), Brazil

Prachi M Desai
Department of Oral Medicine and Radiology, Goa Dental College and Hospital, Bambolim, Goa 403202, India

Beatriz Diaz Fabregat
Department of Preventive and Restorative Dentistry, School of Dentistry, Araçatuba, São Paulo State University (Unesp), Brazil

Amir I O Ibrahim
Department of Restorative Dentistry, College of Dentistry, King Faisal University, Saudi Arabia

Ashok Kumar Jena
Department of Dentistry, All India Institute of Medical Sciences, Bhubaneswar, India

Manisha M Khorate
Department of Oral Medicine and Radiology, Goa Dental College and Hospital, Bambolim, Goa 403202, India

Veena Koul
Centre for Biomedical Engineering, Indian Institute of Technology Delhi, New Delhi, India

Sonali Meher
Neural Developmental Biology Lab, Department of Life Science, National Institute of Technology, Rourkela 769008, Odisha, India

Anisha Mishra
Department of Dentistry, All India Institute of Medical Sciences, Bhubaneswar, India

Monalisa Mishra
Neural Developmental Biology Lab, Department of Life Science, National Institute of Technology, Rourkela 769008, Odisha, India

Douglas Roberto Monteiro
Postgraduate Program in Health Sciences, University of Western São Paulo (UNOESTE), 19050-920 Presidente Prudente/São Paulo, Brazil

Desigar Moodley
Chief Scientific Officer, Edelweiss Dentistry Products GmbH, Wolfurt, Austria

Evelyn Carmo Oliveira
Department of Preventive and Restorative Dentistry, School of Dentistry, Araçatuba, São Paulo State University (Unesp), Brazil

Juliano Pelim Pessan
Department of Preventive and Restorative Dentistry, School of Dentistry, Araçatuba, São Paulo State University (Unesp), Brazil

Abdul Rohman
Department of Pharmaceutical Chemistry, Faculty of Pharmacy, Universitas Gadjah Mada, Yogyakarta 55281, Indonesia
Center of Excellence, Institute for Halal Industry and Systems (PUI-PT IHIS), Universitas Gadjah Mada, Yogyakarta 55281, Indonesia

Caio Sampaio
Department of Preventive and Restorative Dentistry, School of Dentistry, Araçatuba, São Paulo State University (Unesp), Brazil

Jitendra Sharan
Department of Dentistry, All India Institute of Medical Sciences, Bhubaneswar, India

Regina Titi Christinawati Tandelilin
Faculty of Dentistry, Universitas Gadjah Mada, Yogyakarta 55281, Indonesia

Aniket Vaidya
Department of Oral Medicine and Radiology, Goa Dental College and Hospital, Bambolim, Goa 403202, India

Kushal Yadav
Neural Developmental Biology Lab, Department of Life Science, National Institute of Technology, Rourkela 769008, Odisha, India

Chapter 1

Molecular spectroscopy as an analytical tool for the detection of oral cancer

Abdul Rohman and Regina Titi Christinawati Tandelilin

Oral cancer is the eighth most common cancer worldwide. It represents a significant disease burden; therefore, it is necessary to develop noninvasive methods for the early detection of cancer. Due to the large amount of information produced by molecular spectroscopy, chemometrics or multivariate data analysis is used to process the large data sets obtained from the spectra. Some spectroscopic techniques, including infrared and Raman spectroscopy (RS), combined with classification chemometrics, such as principal component analysis (PCA), hierarchical cluster analysis (HCA), and linear/partial least-squares discriminant analysis, are very effective and efficient for the classification and discrimination of healthy individuals from patients with oral cancers.

1.1 Introduction

Oral cancer (OC) is a serious health problem in some regions of the world. OC has sustainedly increased in Southeast Asian countries because of the common use of tobacco products and betel nut products. Oral cancer is the eighth most common cancer worldwide and represents a significant disease burden. If detected at an early stage, the survival rate for oral cancer is better than 90% at five years, whereas the survival of patients presenting with late-stage disease is only 30%. The five-year survival rate for oral cancer has remained at less than 50% over the last 50 years, since most oral cancers (60%) are diagnosed in their advanced stages (stages III and IV) [1]. Therefore, early detection using a simple and reliable analytical method is very urgent. Annual reports have indicated that 127 000 deaths have occurred because of this disease and the estimated number of new cases is 263 000 worldwide. In the United States, 24 000 new cases and 5500 deaths occur due to oral cancers annually [2]. Oral cancers are malignant growths in the human mouth, and they are considered to be life-threatening if they are not correctly diagnosed and treated in

doi:10.1088/978-0-7503-5316-8ch1

their early stages. Oral squamous cell carcinoma (OSCC) is reported to be the most common type of oral cancer [3].

Some techniques used for the diagnosis of oral cancer include physical examination, histopathological examination, vital staining techniques, biopsy, imaging techniques, magnetic resonance imaging, spectroscopic methods, and others, as compiled in figure 1.1 [4]. Some factors contributing to the delayed diagnosis of patients with oral cancer include the lack of effective and efficient tools intended for the screening of oral cancer, insufficient patient education, some difficulties encountered during the risk evaluation of malignant transformation in oral malignant lesions, and the high degree of return following treatment [5]. For these reasons, the early detection of oral cancer is very urgent. The current gold standard method for the diagnosis of suspicious lesions is biopsy and subsequent histopathological evaluation under a microscope. This process is invasive, time-consuming, and subject to interobserver variability [6]. In addition, histopathological tests of biopsied materials and the assessment of the results inevitably cause a diagnostic delay, thus simple methods based on spectroscopic measurements to accurately diagnose tissue pathology without the need for biopsy are continuously being developed [7]. Numerous molecular spectroscopic techniques based on the interaction of photons or electromagnetic radiation with certain molecules in oral cancers have been proposed and developed for the detection of oral cancer, including elastic scattering spectroscopy, elastic light single-scattering spectroscopy [7], fluorescence, diffuse reflectance spectroscopy [8], RS [9], and infrared spectroscopy [10], especially combined with multivariate data analysis. Some of these techniques are used as diagnostic methods and for the early recognition and detection of oral cancer.

Molecular spectroscopy techniques including ultraviolet–visible (UV–vis), fluorescence, infrared (IR), and nuclear magnetic resonance (NMR) have been widely

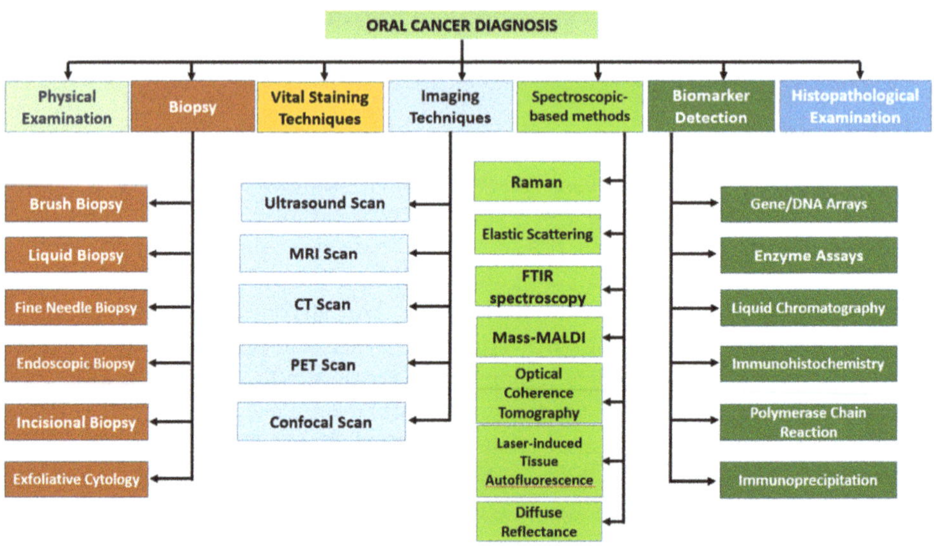

Figure 1.1. Some techniques typically used for oral cancer detection. Adapted from [4] © 2020 with permission from The Authors. Production and hosting by Elsevier B.V. on behalf of KeAi Communications Co., Ltd..

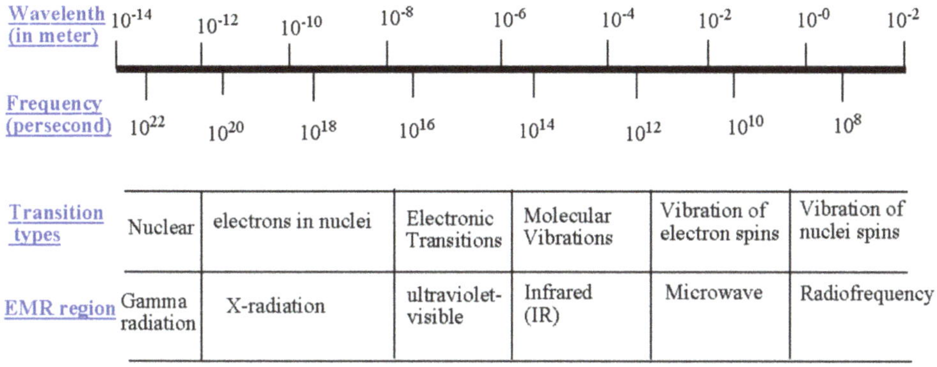

Figure 1.2. The wavelengths, transition types, and EMR regions typically applied in spectroscopic methods. Adapted from [12]. John Wiley & Sons. Copyright © 2011 Wiley-VCH Verlag GmbH & Co. KGaA.

employed for the quality control of medicinal products and as diagnostic tools for certain diseases. All spectroscopic measurements are based on the interaction between electromagnetic radiation (EMR) at a certain wavelength, frequency, or wave number and certain properties of the analytes of interest [11]. Spectroscopic methods are named and applied based on the EMR region involved. UV–vis spectroscopy is based on the interaction between the ultraviolet and visible regions of the electromagnetic spectrum corresponding to wavelengths of 200–380/400 nm and analytes; this causes electronic transitions to take place from the ground state into the singlet excited state. Mid-IR and RS use wave numbers of 400–4000 cm^{-1} to create vibrational transitions in the functional groups in molecules [12]. The wavelengths, transition types, and EMR regions typically applied in spectroscopic methods are depicted in figure 1.2.

The molecular spectra obtained can be used as qualitative and quantitative information for certain analytical tasks; this includes their use in diagnostic tools. Some spectra, especially vibrational spectroscopy spectra (IR, Raman, and NMR), exhibit fingerprint profiles and are useful for differentiating between samples from different classes (for example, in order to discriminate healthy individuals from oral cancer patients). Molecular spectra are also useful for quantitative analyses based on the Beer–Lambert law, according to which the absorbance values of molecular spectra are proportional to their concentrations in objects (samples) [13]. The quantities of data obtained during molecular spectroscopic measurements are very large, which makes it difficult to extract understandable information from them. Fortunately, the special statistics tool called chemometrics can address this obstacle [14].

1.2 Chemometrics

Chemometrics or multivariate data analysis (MDA), also known as artificial intelligence, involves the use of large data sets. In other words, chemometrics deals with the analysis of big data. Chemometrics is typically defined as the employment of statistical and mathematical applications to treat chemical data obtained from analytical measurements [15, 16]. The chemical data subjected to chemometric analyses are not limited to quantitative data such as concentrations; in some cases, chemometrics is used to treat qualitative data such as the colors of samples [17]. In oral diagnostics, some of the chemometrics techniques applied to treat chemical data obtained from molecular spectroscopic measurements include spectral preprocessing, classification using unsupervised pattern recognition, and classification using supervised pattern recognition, as shown in figure 1.3 [18].

Before chemometric analysis takes place, molecular spectra are subjected to spectral preprocessing that is suitable for the intended purpose. The preprocessing of molecular spectral data has become an essential part of chemometric modeling. The preprocessing of spectral data aims to remove physical phenomena from the spectra in order to improve the subsequent chemometric application (e.g. exploratory analysis, a classification model, or multivariate calibration). Most of the preprocessing methods widely employed for molecular spectra can be divided into two groups, namely: (1) scatter-correction methods, which include multiplicative scatter correction (MSC), extended MSC, inverse MSC, extended inverse MSC, de-trending, standard normal variate (SNV), and normalization and (2) spectral derivatives, which include Norris–Williams (NW) and Savitzky–Golay (SG) polynomial derivatives. Both preprocessing methods may apply spectral smoothing before calculating the spectral derivative in an attempt to decrease the detrimental effects on the signal-to-noise ratio [19]. Regardless of the type of preprocessing, the objective of this action is to enhance a subsequent exploratory analysis or pattern recognition, to improve a subsequent classification model, or to enhance the usability of multivariate calibrations for quantitative modeling [20].

Among the chemometric techniques, chemometric models intended for classification or pattern recognition are the most common. The chemometric classification methods focus on the possibility of assigning an object (sample) to a class based on

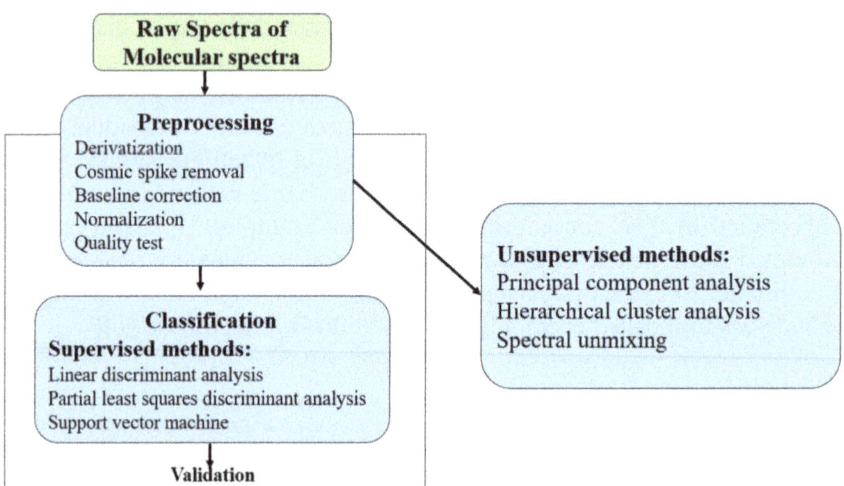

Figure 1.3. Typical chemometric techniques employed in oral diagnostics. Adapted from [18] (2015), reprinted by permission of the publisher (Taylor & Francis Ltd, http://www.tandfonline.com.)

the result of a set of variables obtained from chemical measurements [21, 22]. PCA and HCA are sometimes referred as unsupervised pattern recognition; they are widely employed with classification models for objects (samples). Both chemometric techniques are mainly applied for exploratory purposes, to identify trends, and to find the similarities and differences among samples by reducing the data dimensionality and also to extract the dominant patterns from complex data matrices [23]. The objective of PCA is to find the so-called principal components (PCs), which are linear combinations of the original variables. PCs are sometimes called score plots and referred to as latent variables, since objects with the sample score plot (or PC) values have the same properties in terms of the variables used. Therefore, PCs, as the output of PCA, are employed for the classification and differentiation of objects [24]. Furthermore, HCA is based on the measurement of Euclidean distance; it is typically applied for the clustering of objects. In addition, HCA is an effective tool for detecting hidden correlations between variables [25]. Both chemometric techniques are applied extensively for the classification of healthy individuals and cancer patients using variables of absorbance values obtained from molecular spectroscopic measurements [26–28].

The chemometric models used in supervised pattern recognition employ chemical data (i.e. the responses obtained from molecular spectroscopic measurements) to find the memberships of known classes (groups) of objects (samples). These chemometric models provide a rule that is used to assign new samples to certain classes. First, training models with known classes of objects are developed and validated. The training models are then used to assign new objects into predefined classes in training sets [29]. From an operational point of view, the supervised classification models can be further subdivided into discriminant models and class models. Some discriminant models, including linear discriminant analysis (LDA), partial least-squares discriminant analysis (PLS-DA), orthogonal projections to latent structures discriminant analysis (OPLS-DA), and *k*-nearest neighbors (*k*-NN) focus on finding the differences between samples belonging to different groups [28]. In addition, class modeling based on soft independent modeling of class analogy (SIMCA) and unequal class modeling (UNEQ) focuses on finding the similarities between samples (objects) in the same group; thus, the class modeling decides whether a new sample belongs to a certain group or not [30].

Chemometric classification or pattern recognition models can be selected based on their characteristics, the data structure, and the intended use. It is difficult to provide decision rules for the selection of particular models, an activity that has become a matter of trial and error. However, some tips can be used based on a knowledge of the data structure. For the instance, if a linear relationship is observed between the variables (absorbance values of molecular spectra) and class indexes, then PCA or other linear models are beneficial for the classification of objects. LDA and PLS-DA are considered to be ideal classification chemometrics models for classifying and discriminating between objects (samples) if the variability within a group of objects is greater than that between some groups. In addition, if the relationship between variables and the class index is nonlinear, then a nonlinear discrimination model, such as a quadratic model, or another nonlinear model, such as an artificial neural network (ANN), should be employed [31]. This classification model is popularly used in medical modeling applications [32].

1.3 Fluorescence spectroscopy

Synchronous luminescence spectroscopy (SLS) provides specific and sensitive methods for the identification of certain components used as biological markers in oral cancers. SLS combined with LDA has been employed for the characterization and differentiation of oral cancer tissue. Spectral processing using a deconvolution method has been employed to scan and compute the intensities of fluorescence, peak wavelength, and full width at half maximum for different endogenous fluorophores. During this study, fluorescence measurements were taken from 21 normal and 88 oral squamous cell carcinoma biopsy tissues. The SL spectra of normal and oral cancer tissues exhibit some emission peaks centered at wavelengths of 300, 350, 440, 530, and 630 nm, which are correlated with tryptophan, collagen, nicotinamide adenine dinucleotide (NADH), flavin adenine dinucleotide (FAD), and porphyrin, respectively. A difference between normal and oral cancer tissues could be seen in the spectral changes at these wavelengths. In addition, peak shifts and peak broadening are seen in tryptophan, NADH, and FAD in oral cancer tissues, indicating that either biochemical or environmental changes have taken place at a cellular level. LDA showed that oral cancer tissue can be discriminated from normal tissue with a sensitivity and specificity of 100% and 95.2%, respectively. This confirmed that the combination of SLS and LDA provides an effective and fast method for discriminating between normal and oral cancer tissues [33].

Two molecular spectroscopies, namely fluorescence spectroscopy (FS) using an excitation wavelength of 350 nm and Stokes shift spectroscopy (SSS) with a 120 nm shift have been used to test saliva as a diagnostic medium for the detection of oral cancer. Two chemometrics approaches for pattern recognition, namely PCA and LDA, were applied for the discrimination and classification of three groups: OSCC, oral sub-mucous fibrosis (OSMF) (precancer), and healthy controls (normal). During this study, 99 saliva samples were tested and subjected to spectral measurements using FS and SSS. PCA was used to determine the number of PCs in the spectral data of FS and SSS. The first four PCs (PC1 to PC4) of FS and the first six PCs (PC1 to PC6) of SSS were adopted for classification modeling using LDA with a variance of $\geqslant 98\%$. The scores of LDA using fluorescence spectra as a variable in a spectral range of 380–650 nm with 350 nm excitation were capable of classifying normal and OSCC samples, normal and OSMF samples, and OSCC and OSMF samples with sensitivities of 91, 92, and 91% and specificities of 97%, 100%, and 94%, respectively. In addition, LDA scores obtained using SSS spectra as a variable with a 120 nm Stokes shift in the spectral range of 250–550 nm were capable of discriminating between the respective groups with sensitivities of 100%, 94%, and 94% and specificities of 97%, 100%, and 94%, respectively. Cross-validation using the leave-one-out technique based on data sets of the PC scores showed that both the sensitivity and specificity of the SSS data were less affected than those of the FS data. This study showed that saliva could be used as a potential noninvasive and simple diagnostic method for the detection of oral cancers. Furthermore, SSS provided better diagnostic tools than FS for oral precancer [27].

1.4 Infrared spectroscopy

As for other types of molecular spectroscopy, IR spectroscopy is based on the interaction between EMR in the infrared regions and the functional groups in molecules, which creates vibrational transitions. When a molecule is irradiated by IR radiation, the functional groups in the molecules absorb a certain amount of the incident radiation corresponding to wave numbers at a specific energy, which causes the bonds of the molecules to undergo vibrational excitation into a vibrational energy state. The unique fingerprint patterns of IR absorption caused by particular functional groups produce characteristic bands in their Fourier-transform infrared spectroscopy (FTIR) spectra. Based on Hooke's law, the positions of the peaks and shoulders that represent the absorption of IR radiation by functional groups are affected by the mass that is vibrating, the strength of the molecular bond, the intra- and inter-molecular environment, and the coupling of the fundamental vibrations with other vibrations [34, 35]. Furthermore, the peak intensity (peak height) is proportional to the concentration of the corresponding chemical moieties, which can be further used for quantitative analysis according to the Beer–Lambert law [36]. When combined with MDA or chemometrics, FTIR spectroscopy is a powerful method for differentiating between healthy individuals and cancer patients [37].

Infrared spectroscopy, either in the near-IR (NIR) corresponding to wave numbers in the region of 12 500–4000 cm^{-1}, the mid-IR region at 4000–400 cm^{-1}, or the far region at 400–10 cm^{-1} offers fingerprinting techniques for the characterization and discrimination of objects. The most commonly employed IR region for biological applications is the mid-IR region, which includes the fingerprint region at 1800–900 cm^{-1} for nucleic acids (DNA and RNA), proteins (amides I/II/III), lipids and fatty acids, and carbohydrates. The NIR spectra are occupied by overtones or combinations of the fundamental bands observed in the mid-IR region [38]. FTIR spectroscopy provides fingerprint profiles of biochemicals including proteins, nucleic acids, lipids, and carbohydrates in biological samples; the use of such profiles is typically called *biomolecular fingerprinting*. These profiles are sensitive enough to probe subtle changes in the molecular structure and microenvironment, such as the secondary structures of proteins, the mutation of nucleic acids, and the peroxidation of phospholipids [39, 40]. The biomolecular fingerprinting method has been widely applied for the analysis of analytes in biological fluids [41]. IR spectroscopy has been studied extensively for the identification of several types of cancers [42].

Adeeba *et al* developed FTIR spectroscopy in combination with MDA or chemometrics as an easy, rapid, and efficient method for the analysis of plasma samples of OC patients, healthy individuals (HIs), and tobacco users in order to obtain a picture of OC. Fingerprint profiling of these three groups was carried out in the fingerprint region of the attenuated total reflection (ATR)-FTIR spectra at wave numbers of 1500–500 cm^{-1}. In this study, 147 plasma samples taken from 67 OC patients, 60 tobacco users, and 20 HI controls were subjected to ATR-FTIR spectral measurements. In the FTIR spectral investigation, the height ratios of two peaks at wave numbers of 1646 and 1550 cm^{-1} due to the stretching vibrations of amide I and amide II (A_{1646}/A_{1550}), at wave numbers of 1080 cm^{-1} due to the vibrations of C–O in DNA and RNA, and at 1024 cm^{-1} due to the vibration of the out-of-plane C–O–O–C of DNA and RNA (A_{1080}/A_{1024}) provided differentiation between OC, HI control, and tobacco user samples with p-values of 2.01×10^{-6} and 8.39×10^{-7}, respectively. Three chemometrics, namely PCA, PLS-DA, and OPLS-DA were used to perform the classification between the groups (OC patients, HI controls, and tobacco users). PCA was employed to obtain the separation tendency of all objects in the same group. During PCA, ten samples appeared to be strong outliers and exceeded Hotelling's 99% confidence limit; therefore, these ten samples were removed. The OPLS-DA model offered better discrimination than PLS-DA for the three groups, achieving sensitivity, specificity, and classification rates of 99.9%, 98%, and 89.7% (OPLS-DA) compared to 97.9%, 97%, and 87.5% (PLS-DA), respectively. This study confirmed that the combination of ATR-FTIR spectra and suitable chemometric classification could provide initial differentiation between plasma samples taken from OC patients, tobacco users, and normal (healthy) individuals effectively and efficiently [43].

The ATR-FTIR spectra of salivary exosomes were acquired from patients with OC and HIs. These spectra, combined with chemometrics based on PCA–LDA and support vector machine (SVM) classification, were assessed for their suitability as a potential diagnostic tool for oral cancer. Samples of whole saliva were obtained from 21 OC patients and 13 HIs. The ATR-FTIR spectra were scanned at wave numbers of 900–5000 cm^{-1}. The characteristic performances of sensitivity, specificity, and the area under the receiver operating characteristic curve were calculated. The ATR-FTIR spectra of the OC patients were consistently different from those of HIs, especially at wave numbers of 1072 cm^{-1} (due to nucleic acids), 2924 cm^{-1} and 2854 cm^{-1} (lipid components), and 1543 cm^{-1} (proteins). Using the chemometric method of PCA–LDA, the discrimination model was able to classify the samples (OC and HI) with a sensitivity, specificity, and accuracy of 100%, 89%, and of 95%, respectively. In addition, SVM achieved a classification model accuracy of 100% (in the training model) and an accuracy of 89% (in the cross-validation model), indicating that the combination of ATR-FTIR spectra and chemometrics (PCA–LDA and SVM) is an effective analytical method for oral cancer detection [28].

FTIR spectroscopy coupled with the classification chemometrics of a quadratic support vector machine (SVM) was developed and validated to discriminate between oral leukoplakia (OLK) and OSCC. This study scanned the FTIR spectra of paraffin-embedded tissue taken from 47 human subjects (eight HIs, 16 OLK patients, and 23 OSCC patients). The spectral preprocessing included difference between mean spectra (DBMS). The Mann–Whitney's test and forward feature selection (FFS) models were applied during the optimization and selection of FTIR spectra as the spectral marker. Classification chemometrics of linear SVM and quadratic SVM (with tenfold cross-validation using different combinations of spectral features) were used for the classification of normal, OLK, and OSCC samples. Using six features obtained through FFS, it was possible to discriminate between normal and OSCC tissues, in which the peaks at wave numbers of 1782, 1713, 1665, 1545, 1409, and 1161 cm^{-1} provided the greatest contributions. The developed model was also successful in discriminating and classifying OLK and OSCC, achieving a sensitivity of 81.3% and a specificity of 95.7% with an overall accuracy of 89.7% [10]. This result indicated that the combination of FTIR spectra and SVM is a specific and accurate tool for the discrimination and classification of normal, OLK, and OSCC samples.

1.5 Raman spectroscopy

RS is a type of vibrational spectroscopy that is widely applied for the detection of oral cancers. This technique is complementary to infrared spectroscopy. RS detects molecular vibration information by collecting the light produced by inelastic scattering, which allows the 'fingerprint properties' of a sample to be acquired [44]. RS offers some advantages for oral diagnostics, namely: (1) RS can be employed with a large range of biomedical samples, including single fibers, crystals, films, suspensions, and precipitates; (2) RS needs minimum sample preparation and in some cases no fixation or staining; (3) RS offers a high degree of accuracy and precision; (4) RS requires a minimum amount of the sample compared to other diagnostic techniques; (5) RS is considered to be a nondestructive and noninvasive analytical method for medical applications in which the samples measured with RS could be analyzed using other analytical methods; and (6) the spectra of RS can be obtained quickly [9]. However, some disadvantages related to RS are also encountered, namely: (1) a weak signal is obtained, especially for samples with polar functional groups, due to the produced Raman effect; (2) RS peaks typically overlap, which creates some difficulties for the identification of individual components present in the evaluated samples; (3) the peaks obtained during RS measurements are typically numerous and require sophisticated data treatments [18, 41]. Some reviews have been published that describe the application of RS and chemometrics in oral diagnostics [18, 44, 45].

RS in combination with chemometrics based on PCA has been applied to differentiate and classify HIs and patients with malignant epithelial cells with the objective of detecting oral cancer. A detailed investigation revealed that some drastic changes in Raman spectra can be observed between the two groups (HIs and patients with oral cancers), especially at wave numbers of 1470, 1280, 1240, 1100–1050 cm^{-1}, and around 850 cm^{-1}. These spectral differences between normal and malignant patients seem to arise from compositional differences in proteins or changes in the conformations or structures of proteins. In addition, the protein content is increased in malignant epithelia compared to normal cells. Furthermore, PCA using all absorbance values in the Raman spectra as variables was able to classify epithelial normal, epithelial malignant, sub-epithelial normal, and sub-epithelial malignant cells. This result indicated that the combination of micro-Raman spectra and PCA could be an effective tool for the screening for oral cancers based on the detection of malignant epithelial cells [46]. Raman spectra were also accurately reported to predict disease-free survival (DFS) in oral squamous carcinoma using the spectral region of 1200–1800 cm^{-1} [47]. Using an appropriate selection of wave numbers and peak intensities in the Raman spectra, it was easy to differentiate and classify normal and abnormal conditions due to oral cancers.

The potential use of *in vivo* RS in combination with multivariate data analysis has been proposed for the diagnosis of malignant and potentially malignant lesions of the human oral cavity in a clinical setting. This study involved 28 healthy volunteers and 171 patients with various lesions of the oral cavity. The Raman spectra were scanned at multiple sites of normal oral mucosa and lesions belonging to three histopathological categories, namely OSCC, OSMF, and OLK. The Raman spectra obtained were subjected to a probability-based multivariate statistical algorithm capable of direct multiclass classification via a maximum representation and discrimination feature (MRDF) and probabilistic classification via sparse multinomial logistic regression (SMLR). Using MRDF, SMLR, and cross-validation based on the leave-one-out technique, the accuracy values obtained were 85%, 89%, 85% and 82% for the classifications of four groups (control, OSCC, OSMF, and OLK), respectively. The accuracy rates were increased when MRDF–SMLR was used for the classification of normal versus malignant samples (sensitivity 96%, specificity 99%), normal versus potentially malignant samples (sensitivity 99%, specificity 98%), and normal versus abnormal samples (sensitivity and specificity of 94%). This result was confirmed using the standard method of histological investigation [48]. Raman spectra were also successfully employed for the identification of sequential progression in experimental oral carcinogenesis in a model of the hamster buccal pouch through three approaches, namely *ex vivo*, *in vivo* sequential, and *in vivo* follow-up. Changes of the Raman spectra were observed in the early stages as the lipid components dominated, while increased levels of the protein-to-lipid ratio and nucleic acids were observed in the later stages and in tumors. This confirms that the differences in Raman spectra are associated with the different levels of biocomponents present at each stage of oral carcinogenesis [49].

Ultrasensitive surface-enhanced Raman scattering (SERS) based on gold nanoparticles in combination with the unsupervised pattern recognition of PCA has been applied for the detection and diagnosis of oral cancer by analyzing the saliva of patients, since saliva contains abundant proteins and metabolites which can indicate the health status of an individual. Saliva is also an optimal sample for noninvasive cancer detection. During the scanning of SERS spectra, some changes in terms of the variability of signal intensities and frequency shifts were observed in oral cancer samples versus healthy saliva. Based on PCA, the healthy saliva could be discriminated and classified from oral cancer saliva using a variable that represented several SERS peaks assigned mainly to amino acids and proteins. Based on a loading plot of the PCA, the cancer group displayed a high-intensity peak at a wave number of 2126 cm^{-1}, which corresponds to the stretching vibrations of C–N in thiocyanate [50]. Furthermore, some SERS marker bands that contributed to the discrimination between healthy and oral cancer saliva were located at wave numbers of 1612 cm^{-1} (due to lipid components), 1414 cm^{-1} (fatty acids), 1403 cm^{-1} (nucleic acids), 1336, 1259, and 1072 cm^{-1} due to amino acids such as tyrosine, tryptophan, and proteins and 738 cm cm^{-1} (thiocyanate) [51]. The combination of SERS and the score plot obtained from PCA could be an effective tool for the classification of normal and oral cancer saliva, while the loading plot obtained via PCA could offer the peaks that provide the greatest differentiation between normal and oral cancer saliva.

Two vibrational spectroscopies, namely Raman and FTIR spectroscopy, were employed in combination with chemometric techniques (PCA, LDA) for the classification and discrimination of normal, precancerous, and cancerous conditions. This study investigated 13 HIs, 13 precancer patients, and 10 cancer patients. Samples of oral exfoliated cells were collected and subjected to FTIR and Raman spectral measurements. In this detailed investigation, some peaks contributed more to the differentiation between the three classes, namely wave numbers of 1550 cm^{-1}, 1580, 1640, 2370, 2330, 2950–3000, and 3650–3750 cm^{-1} (in the FTIR spectra) and wave numbers of 520 cm^{-1}, 640, 785, 827, 850, 935, 1003, 1175, 1311, and 1606 cm^{-1} (in the Raman spectra). The combination of PCA–LDA, the use of tenfold cross-validation, and the application of the absorbance values of the FTIR spectra and the Raman spectral data sets yielded efficient classification and discrimination between normal, precancerous, and cancerous conditions. Using the data fusion of Raman and FTIR spectra, the PCA–LDA accuracy rate obtained was 98%. This accuracy was higher than the accuracy achieved using FTIR spectra alone, which offered an accuracy rate of 85%, or Raman spectra as a variable, which achieved an accuracy level of 82%. Furthermore, the efficiency rates of the classifications were 73%, 80%, and 87% for the variables of the FTIR spectra, the Raman spectra and the data fusion of the Raman and FTIR spectra, respectively. According to the efficiency and accuracy rates, the data fusion of the FTIR and Raman spectra coupled with the PCA–LDA model forms an effective method for the classification of healthy individuals and patients with precancerous and oral cancer conditions. This approach could be extrapolated to detect the oral conditions of non-smoking and smoking patients [26].

List of abbreviations

ANN	Artificial neural networks
DBMS	Difference between mean spectra
LDA	Linear discriminant analysis
MRDF	Maximum representation and discrimination feature ()
MSC	Multiplicative scatter correction
OSCC	Oral squamous cell carcinoma
OSMF	Oral sub-mucous fibrosis
PCA	Principal component analysis
SIMCA	Soft independent modeling of class analogy
SMLR	Sparse multinomial logistic regression
SNV	Standard normal variate
SVM	Support vector machine
UNEQ	Unequal class modeling

References

[1] Omar E 2015 Current concepts and future of noninvasive procedures for diagnosing oral squamous cell carcinoma: a systematic review *Head Face Med* **11**

[2] Wong B J F and Ilgner J 2016 Biomedical optics in otorhinolaryngology: head and neck surgery *Biomed. Opt. Otorhinolaryngol. Head Neck Surg.* 1–653

[3] Kim D H, Kim S W and Hwang S H 2021 Efficacy of non-invasive diagnostic methods in the diagnosis and screening of oral cancer and precancer *Braz. J. Otorhinolaryngol.* **88** 937–47

[4] Borse V, Konwar A N and Buragohain P 2020 Oral cancer diagnosis and perspectives in India *Sens. Int.* **1** 100046

[5] Lingen M W, Kalmar J R, Karrison T and Speight P M 2008 Critical evaluation of diagnostic aids for the detection of oral cancer *Oral Oncol.* **44** 22

[6] Leoncini E *et al* 2014 Adult height and head and neck cancer: a pooled analysis within the INHANCE Consortium *Head Neck* **36** 1391

[7] Sircan-Kucuksayan A, Yaprak N, Derin A T, Ozbudak İ H, Turhan M and Canpolat M 2020 Noninvasive assessment of oral lesions using elastic light single-scattering spectroscopy: a pilot study *Eur. Arch. Oto-Rhino-Laryngology* **277** 1467–72

[8] Bigio I J and Bown S G 2004 Spectroscopic sensing of cancer and cancer therapy: current status of translational research *Cancer Biol. Ther.* **3** 259–67

[9] Alqhtani N, Nhembe F, Upile T and Hopper C 2009 Raman spectroscopy and oral cancer *Head Neck Oncol.* **1** 5

[10] Banerjee S *et al* 2015 Fourier-transform-infrared-spectroscopy based spectral-biomarker selection towards optimum diagnostic differentiation of oral leukoplakia and cancer *Anal. Bioanal. Chem.* **407** 7935–43

[11] Rohman A, Rawar E A, Sudevi S, Nurrulhidayah A F and Windarsih A 2020 The use of chemometrics in combination with molecular spectroscopic and chromatographic methods for authentication of curcuma species: a review *Food Res.* **4** 1850–8

[12] Breuer D 2007 Molecular spectroscopy in the ultraviolet and visible range *The MAK-Collection for Occupational Health and Safety* (New York: Wiley) pp 1–15

[13] Rohman A and Windarsih A 2020 The application of molecular spectroscopy in combination with chemometrics for halal authentication analysis: a review *Int. J. Mol. Sci.* **21** 1–18

[14] Pollo B J *et al* 2021 Chemometrics, comprehensive two-dimensional gas chromatography and 'omics' sciences: basic tools and recent applications *TrAC Trends Anal. Chem.* **134** 116111

[15] Risoluti R, Gullifa G, Battistini A and Materazzi S 2019 MicroNIR/chemometrics: a new analytical platform for fast and accurate detection of Δ9-tetrahydrocannabinol (THC) in oral fluids *Drug Alcohol Depend.* **205** 107578

[16] Kistenev Y V, Borisov A V, Titarenko M A, Baydik O D and Shapovalov A V 2018 Diagnosis of oral lichen planus from analysis of saliva samples using terahertz time-domain spectroscopy and chemometrics *J. Biomed. Opt.* **23** 1

[17] Sezer B, Apaydin H, Bilge G and Boyaci I H 2018 Coffee arabica adulteration: detection of wheat, corn and chickpea *Food Chem.* **264** 142–8

[18] Eberhardt K, Stiebing C, Matthaüs C, Schmitt M and Popp J 2015 Advantages and limitations of Raman spectroscopy for molecular diagnostics: an update *Expert Rev. Mol. Diagn.* **15** 773–87

[19] Lee L C, Liong C Y and Jemain A A 2017 A contemporary review on data preprocessing (DP) practice strategy in ATR-FTIR spectrum *Chemom. Intell. Lab. Syst.* **163** 64–75

[20] Rinnan Å, van den Berg F and Engelsen S B 2009 Review of the most common pre-processing techniques for near-infrared spectra *TrAC Trends Anal. Chem.* **28** 1201–22

[21] Marini F 2009 Classification Methods in Chemometrics *Curr. Anal. Chem.* **6** 72–9

[22] Arifah M F, Hastuti A A M B and Rohman A 2022 Application of molecular spectroscopy and chemometrics for authentication and quality control of tea (*Camellia sinensis* L.): a review *Indones. J. Pharm.* **33** 555–66

[23] Mazivila S J and Olivieri A C 2018 Chemometrics coupled to vibrational spectroscopy and spectroscopic imaging for the analysis of solid-phase pharmaceutical products: a brief review on non-destructive analytical methods *TrAC Trends Anal. Chem.* **108** 74–87

[24] Jugreet B S, Mahomoodally M F, Sinan K I, Zengin G and Abdallah H H 2020 Chemical variability, pharmacological potential, multivariate and molecular docking analyses of essential oils obtained from four medicinal plants *Ind. Crops Prod.* **150** 112394

[25] Cebi N, Yilmaz M T and Sagdic O 2017 A rapid ATR-FTIR spectroscopic method for detection of sibutramine adulteration in tea and coffee based on hierarchical cluster and principal component analyses *Food Chem.* **229** 517–26

[26] Ghosh A, Raha S, Dey S, Chatterjee K, Roy Chowdhury A and Barui A 2019 Chemometric analysis of integrated FTIR and Raman spectra obtained by non-invasive exfoliative cytology for the screening of oral cancer *Analyst* **144** 1309–25

[27] Kumar P, Singh A, Kumar Kanaujia S and Pradhan A 2018 Human saliva for oral precancer detection: a comparison of fluorescence and Stokes shift spectroscopy *J. Fluoresc.* **28** 419–26

[28] Zlotogorski-Hurvitz A, Dekel B Z, Malonek D, Yahalom R and Vered M 2019 FTIR-based spectrum of salivary exosomes coupled with computational-aided discriminating analysis in the diagnosis of oral cancer *J. Cancer Res. Clin. Oncol.* **145** 685–94

[29] Bagur-González M G, Pérez-Castaño E, Sánchez-Viñas M and Gázquez-Evangelista D 2015 Using the liquid-chromatographic-fingerprint of sterols fraction to discriminate virgin olive from other edible oils *J. Chromatogr.* A **1380** 64–70

[30] Kuswandi B, Putri F K, Gani A A and Ahmad M 2015 Application of class-modelling techniques to infrared spectra for analysis of pork adulteration in beef jerkys *J. Food Sci. Technol.* **52** 7655–68

[31] Chen R C, Dewi C, Huang S W and Caraka R E 2020 Selecting critical features for data classification based on machine learning methods *J. Big Data* **7**

[32] Salari N, Shohaimi S, Najafi F, Nallappan M and Karishnarajah I 2013 Application of pattern recognition tools for classifying acute coronary syndrome: an integrated medical modeling *Theor. Biol. Med. Model.* **10** 1–17

[33] Gnanatheepam E, Kanniyappan U, Dornadula K, Prakasarao A and Singaravelu G 2019 Synchronous luminescence spectroscopy as a tool in the discrimination and characterization of oral cancer tissue *J. Fluoresc.* **29** 361–7

[34] Wang R and Wang Y 2021 Fourier transform infrared spectroscopy in oral cancer diagnosis *Int. J. Mol. Sci.* **22** 1–21

[35] Lin X and Sun D W 2020 Recent developments in vibrational spectroscopic techniques for tea quality and safety analyses *Trends Food Sci. Technol.* **104** 163–76

[36] Rohman A, Arifah F H, Irnawati G, Alam M and Muchtaridi 2020 The application of FTIR spectroscopy and chemometrics for classification of Mangosteen extract and its correlation with alpha-mangostin *J. Appl. Pharm. Sci.* **10** 149–54

[37] Yadav D K, Shaikh S and Rawal R 2021 Oral pre-cancer and oral cancer detection by ATR-FTIR spectrometry using blood serum and multivariate data analysis *Indonesian J. Chemom. Pharm. Anal.* **1** 111–20

[38] Rohman A 2017 The use of infrared spectroscopy in combination with chemometrics for quality control and authentication of edible fats and oils: a review *Appl. Spectrosc. Rev.* **52** 589–604

[39] Kelly J G, Martin-Hirsch P L and Martin F L 2009 Discrimination of base differences in oligonucleotides using mid-infrared spectroscopy and multivariate analysis *Anal. Chem.* **81** 5314–9

[40] Ghimire H, Garlapati C, Janssen E A M, Krishnamurti U, Qin G and Aneja R *et al* 2020 Protein conformational changes in breast cancer sera using infrared spectroscopic analysis *Cancers (Basel)* **12** 1708

[41] Rohman A, Windarsih A, Lukitaningsih E, Rafi M, Betania K and Fadzillah N A 2020 The use of FTIR and Raman spectroscopy in combination with chemometrics for analysis of biomolecules in biomedical fluids: a review *Biomed. Spectrosc. Imaging* **8** 55–71

[42] Bel'skaya L V 2019 Use of IR spectroscopy in cancer diagnosis. a review *J. Appl. Spectrosc.* **86** 187–205

[43] Adeeba *et al* 2018 A comparative profiling of oral cancer patients and high risk niswar users using FT-IR and chemometric analysis *Spectrochim. Acta, Part* A **203** 177–84

[44] Zhang Y, Ren L, Wang Q, Wen Z, Liu C and Ding Y 2022 Raman Spectroscopy: a potential diagnostic tool for oral diseases *Front. Cell. Infect. Microbiol.* **12** 775236

[45] Sahu A and Krishna C M 2017 Optical diagnostics in oral cancer: an update on Raman spectroscopic applications *J. Cancer Res. Ther.* **13** 908–15

[46] Krishna C M *et al* 2004 Micro-Raman spectroscopy for optical pathology of oral squamous cell carcinoma *Appl. Spectrosc.* **58** 1128–35

[47] Bhattacharjee A *et al* 2021 Risk prediction by Raman spectroscopy for disease-free survival in oral cancers *Lasers Med. Sci.* **36** 1691–700

[48] Krishna H, Majumder S K, Chaturvedi P, Sidramesh M and Gupta P K 2014 *In vivo* Raman spectroscopy for detection of oral neoplasia: a pilot clinical study *J. Biophotonics* **7** 690–702

[49] Kumar P, Bhattacharjee T, Ingle A, Maru G and Krishna C M 2016 Raman spectroscopy of experimental oral carcinogenesis: study on sequential cancer progression in Hamster Buccal Pouch Model *Technol. Cancer Res. Treat.* **15** NP60–72

[50] Fălămaş A, Rotaru H and Hedeşiu M 2020 Surface-enhanced Raman spectroscopy (SERS) investigations of saliva for oral cancer diagnosis *Lasers Med. Sci.* **35** 1393–401

[51] Movasaghi Z, Rehman S and Rehman I U 2007 Raman spectroscopy of biological tissues *Appl. Spectrosc. Rev.* **42** 493–541

Chapter 2

Nonionizing, noninvasive diagnostic techniques in endodontics

Anisha Mishra, Jitendra Sharan, Veena Koul and Ashok Kumar Jena

2.1 Introduction

Endodontics is a specialized field of oral health science which is concerned with preventing, intercepting, and treating diseases and injuries of the pulp and associated peri-radicular conditions [1]. Accurate diagnosis of pulp and peri-radicular tissue conditions is critical prior to any intervention. Endodontists use their knowledge, experience, and skill, along with the results of diagnostic tests, to formulate and customize a treatment plan. Since the introduction of x-rays by Wilhelm Röntgen in 1895, x-rays have remained one of the most important diagnostic tools used by endodontists to screen the condition of pulp and periodontal tissues, as they help to provide a better understanding of the location, shape, size, and, more recently, even the 3D spatial relationships of oral facial hard tissue structures. Although ionizing radiation offers the advantage of easier diagnosis, it has its own side effects, such as affecting the human body's external and internal sensitive organs [2, 3]. Over time, the diagnostic approaches used by endodontists have seen dramatic changes, which have been made possible by the advent of newer concepts and technologies. The prime concern of the latest techniques is to minimize or completely eliminate the use of ionizing radiation during the diagnostic process, thus enhancing overall patient safety during the endodontic procedure. Successful treatment requires accurate diagnosis, and these novel methods, most of which are non-radiating and noninvasive, can provide valuable information about the pulp status and the periapical and periodontal conditions of teeth. Various nonionizing and noninvasive diagnostic tools and techniques which are frequently used and newly introduced are illustrated in table 2.1.

doi:10.1088/978-0-7503-5316-8ch2

Table 2.1. An overview of the nonionizing, noninvasive diagnostic techniques used in endodontics.

S. No.	Nonionizing, noninvasive diagnostic technique	Mechanism of action	Indications
1	Pulse oximetry	Based on the Beer–Lambert law, it analyzes the differences in the light absorption spectrum caused by oxy- and deoxyhemoglobin	Determination of pulp vitality and pulp status after traumatic injury
2	Laser Doppler flowmetry (LDF)	Based on the Doppler effect, which explains the shift in frequency as a wave is emitted from an object moving away or towards the observer	Determination of pulp vitality and pulp status after traumatic injury
3	Photoplethysmography	Similar to pulse oximetry but uses a shorter wavelength of light	Determination of pulp vitality and pulp status after traumatic injury
4	Spectrophotometry	– Dual-wavelength visible light at 760 nm and 850 nm filtered and guided through fiber optics – Analyzes the oxygenation changes in the capillary bed of the tissue.	– Can be used for determination of pulp vitality and pulp status after traumatic injury – This diagnostic technique still has no specific tool in dentistry
5	Transmitted laser light	Similar to LDF but uses two probes; the sending probe is on the buccal side and the receiver probe is placed on the palatal side of the teeth	Determination of pulp vitality and pulp status after traumatic injury
6	Surface temperature	Analysis of tooth surface temperature using thermistor tubes	Determination of pulp vitality and pulp status after traumatic injury
7	Electrical pulp testing	Electrical stimulus passes through the tip of the device through a conducting medium along the prisms and tubules of enamel and dentin to the pulp tissue thereby causing ionic changes in the nerve membrane and inducing an action potential at the nodes of Ranvier of the A-delta fibers.	Determination of pulp sensibility status and pulp status after traumatic injury

8	Fiber-optic transillumination (FOTI) and digital fiber-optic transillumination (DIFOTI)	– FOTI uses optic fibers to transilluminate the tooth structures in the interproximal areas to detect incipient carious lesions – DIFOTI incorporates a handpiece, a control panel, an image recording system, and detection software to produce *in vivo* digital images with different projection settings for occlusal and interproximal surfaces	Caries detection and staging
9	Near-infrared light transillumination (NILT)	– Consists of elastic arms containing optical fibers transmitting a near-infrared light source (700 nm and 1500 nm), a USB connection to a computer, software, and a camera system. – The elastic arms are placed near the alveolar process against the roots of the tooth. The light scatters from the occlusal surface which is captured by the sensor and displayed on the computer through the software. – The carious lesions appear darker than the surrounding healthy tissues	Caries detection and staging
10	Optical coherence tomography (OCT)	Utilizes a beam of partially coherent light consisting of near-infrared light waves to create tomographic images by reflecting off microstructures	– Caries detection and staging – Imaging of teeth, periodontal structures, and restorative margins – Identification of vertical root fractures – To avoid inadvertent pulp exposure during tooth preparation – Monitoring of dentin bridge formation for information on the outcome of pulp capping

(*Continued*)

Table 2.1. (*Continued*)

S. No.	Nonionizing, noninvasive diagnostic technique	Mechanism of action	Indications
11	Electrical conductance and impedance	Based on the principle that sound enamel has low percentages of fluid and porosity and is hence a poor conductor of electricity	Caries detection and staging
12	Electrical caries monitor	Uses single-, fixed-frequency alternating current to assess the bulk resistance of the tooth	Caries detection and staging
13	CarieScan Pro	Measures the electrical impedance on a scale	Caries detection and staging
14	DIAGNOdent	Based on laser fluorescence which emits a monochromatic red laser beam at 655 nm, exciting bacterial photoporphyrins, which ultimately results in detectable fluorescence	Caries detection and staging
15	Midwest Caries ID	– Analyzes the translucency and opacity of the tooth micro-structure by determining the mineral content and integrity of enamel rods based on the reflection and refraction of the emitted light from the analyzed surface. – Based on LED technology. It emits light at wavelengths between 635 nm and 880 nm and the emitted light is captured by the fiber optics that converts it into electrical signals for further analysis	Caries detection and staging
16	VistaCam	– Based on intraoral fluorescence; consists of six violet- light-generating LEDs at a wavelength of 405 nm – The camera, when directed at the tooth surface illuminates the surface and captures the reflected light which is filtered for light at less than 495 nm to differentiate healthy teeth from carious lesions	Caries detection and staging

17	Soprolife® System	Consists of two types of LED which illuminate either in the white light region or in a narrow band at a wavelength of 450 nm and a bandwidth of 20 nm	Caries detection and staging
18	SiroInspect	Illuminates the tooth with violet light at a wavelength of 405 nm, which stimulates the decomposition products of the carious dentin, including the healthy tooth structurez	Caries detection and staging
19	Quantitative light- (or laser-) induced fluorescence	– Based on the property of fluorescence which is the emission of light at a higher wavelength after absorbing incident light at a shorter wavelength – As carious activity progresses into the dentin, the incident light scatters more and hence the fluorescence is reduced	Caries detection and staging
20	Photothermal radiometry and modulated luminescence	Consists of modulated thermal infrared radiation and alternating-current luminescence	Caries detection and staging
21	Electronic apex locator	– Electrical resistance between the mucous membrane and the periodontal structures is 6 kΩ – With the advancement of the file into the canal, the circuit is completed and the resistance between the file and mucosa is equalized; a signal is visualized confirming that the file is at the apex	– Locating tooth apex – Detecting root perforations, fractures, and cracks and internal or external resorption

(*Continued*)

Table 2.1. (*Continued*)

S. No.	Nonionizing, noninvasive diagnostic technique	Mechanism of action	Indications
22	Magnetic resonance imaging (MRI)	– Hydrogen protons spin about their axes and when the patient is placed in a magnetic field, the nuclei align to the direction of the magnetic field. – When a radio-frequency wave is sent, it impacts all the hydrogen protons and alters their movement from the longitudinal to the transverse plane. – On stoppage of the radio-frequency signal, the nuclei lose energy and return to their equilibrium longitudinal axes, giving off a measurable signal.	– Detection of odontogenic cysts and tumors – Longitudinal evaluation of teeth treated with regenerative procedures – Understanding root canal anatomy – Crack detection – Pulp vitality, pulp regeneration/ reperfusion, stem-cell-based regeneration assessment – Endodontic treatment prediction
23	Ultrasound imaging	– Based on the reflections and echoes of sound waves; employs a transducer which transmits high-frequency pulses in the range of 1–20 MHz. – On returning to the transducer, the waves differ on a gray scale based on the density of the tissues	– Evaluation of hard and soft dental tissues – Measurement of pulpal blood flow to determine pulp vitality – Aid in the accurate diagnosis and differentiation of periapical lesions – Monitor healing of lesions of endodontic origin – Caries and crack detection – Sinus tracing

2.2 Pulpal status diagnosis

2.2.1 Pulp vitality assessment

2.2.1.1 Pulse oximetry

The pulse oximeter works using the principle of the Beer–Lambert law by analyzing the different light absorbance spectra of oxy- and deoxyhemoglobin. The law states that 'an unknown concentration of solute (hemoglobin) dissolved in a known solvent (blood) can be assessed by the light absorption of the solute' [4, 5].

The probe consists of two light-emitting diodes; one produces red light (660 nm) to measure the absorption of oxygenated hemoglobin and the other produces infrared light (900–940 nm) to measure deoxygenated hemoglobin [6–12]. A photodetector diode connected to a microprocessor receives the light, and the relationship between the pulsatile changes in absorption rates of the two lights ultimately shows the oxygen saturation (SpO2) of the arterial blood (figure 2.1). This accurately diagnoses pulpal inflammation and necrosis and, in turn, vitality.

Although recent meta-analyses of the diagnostic accuracy of pulp tests have shown pulp oximetry to be the most accurate compared to other tests, it still has its limitations. Currently, no oximeters are made especially for dentistry due to the challenge of keeping both diodes parallel, as minor movements can alter the results [14, 15]. Trials of custom-made probes with parallel sensors have been attempted by a few authors [13, 16, 17]. Additional factors, such as the surrounding structures and their differing morphologies that scatter light in different ways, transmitter light power, ambient light, restorative materials, and prostheses can alter the readings' accuracy [18]. Moreover, time-dependant, morphophysiological changes that occur

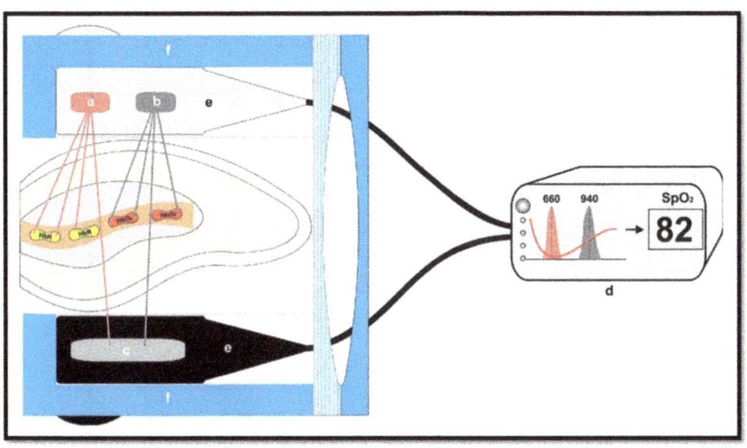

Figure 2.1. The operaational mechanism of the dental pulse oximeter. (a) A light-emitting diode emitting red light at 660 nm, (b) a light-emitting diode emitting infrared light at 940 nm, (c) a photodetector, (d) a pulse oximeter monitor, (e) a pulse oximeter sensor, (f) a custom-made pulse oximeter sensor holder. HbO_2, oxygenated hemoglobin; HbR, deoxygenated hemoglobin; SpO_2, oxygen saturation of arterial blood. Reprinted from [13], Copyright (2007), with permission from Elsevier and the American Association of Endodontists.

in the pulp–dentin complex with age, such as the deposition of mineralized tissue, can also hinder the dispersion of light, thereby altering the reading [19].

2.2.1.2 Laser Doppler flowmetry

Laser Doppler flowmetry is based on the Doppler effect described by Christian Doppler [20] (figure 2.2), which explains the shift in frequency that occurs as a wave is emitted from an object moving away from or towards the observer. A fiber-optic probe that transmits two equal-intensity laser light beams (one from a He–Ne laser at 632.8 nm and the other from a semiconductor laser at 780–820 nm) [21] is focused on the tooth surface. Moving red blood cells scatter the light beams and shift the frequency; hence, the reflected light is returned to the afferent fiber through the same probe to the photodetectors, creating a signal [22–26].

The output signal, also termed the 'flux,' is the number of moving red blood cells per second times their mean velocities [28]. When the signals obtained from vital and non-vital pulp are compared, the flux is always higher in the former compared to the latter [29]. Flowmetry can also detect changes in the optical properties of necrotic teeth.

However, it is advisable to interpret the values obtained with care, as they can be ambiguous and semi-quantitative [30]. The device is also susceptible to external noises, vibrations, movements, and blood flow in proximate tissues. Another major limitation is that the device only detects coronal pulpal blood flow, which results in

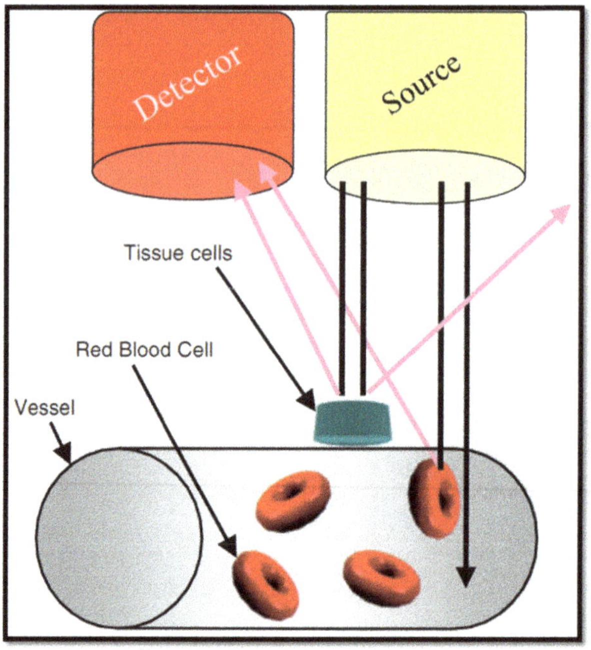

Figure 2.2. The application of the Doppler principle in laser Doppler flowmetry [27] John Wiley & Sons. (License No. 5482930328720).

mineralized tissues of varying thickness; the presence of restorative materials can alter the signals produced [31].

2.2.1.3 Photoplethysmography

Transmitted-light photoplethysmography is an optical measurement technique that aids pulpal vitality assessment in a similar way to pulse oximetry but uses a shorter wavelength of light. It consists of a light source and a photodetector that measures the perfusion and volumetric changes in the pulp microvasculature. The hemoglobin in the pulp absorbs certain wavelengths of light; the remaining light is scattered through the tooth and picked up by the photodetector. The resultant waveforms are pulsatile and synchronous with a finger photoplethysmography reference (figure 2.3). Hence, loss of pulsatility indicates non-vitality of the pulp. The advantage of this method over laser Doppler flowmetry is that the surrounding periodontal blood flow has lower signal contamination effects on the obtained results [32–37].

2.2.1.4 Spectrophotometry

Spectrophotometry utilizes dual-wavelength visible light at 760 nm and 850 nm that is filtered and guided through fiber optics. It analyzes oxygenation changes in the capillary bed of the tissue rather than the supply vessels, which makes it independent of the pulsatile circulation. In an *in vitro* study, Nissan *et al* found that continuous wave spectrophotometry could be an adjunctive tool for pulp vitality testing when comparing teeth with empty pulp chambers, chambers filled with fixed pulp tissue, or oxygenated blood. There is still no specific spectrophotometric tool designed for dental purposes [38].

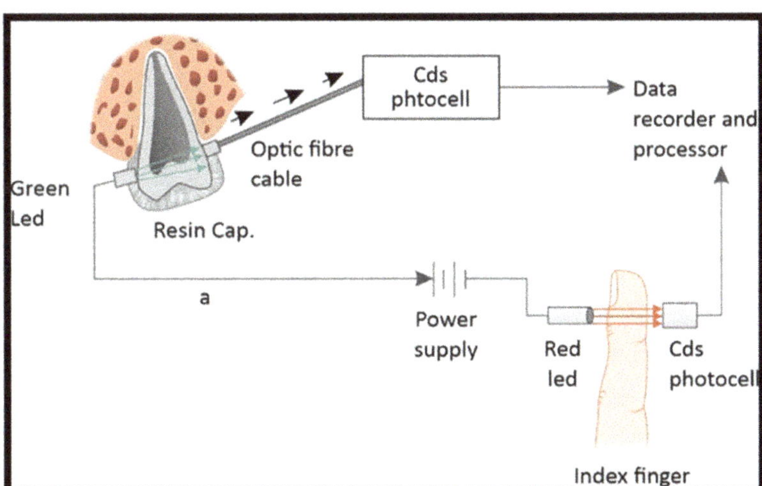

Figure 2.3. The mechanism of transmitted-light photoplethysmography and finger photoplethysmography.

2.2.1.5 Transmitted laser light

Laser Doppler flowmetry has the disadvantages of recording even non-pulpal signals and wrongly assessing non-vital teeth with recordings greater than zero. This may be attributed to positioning the device near the enamel surface, which causes interference and backscattering of light due to the blood flow in the surrounding tissues. Hence, transmitted laser light was an experimental variation that used two probes: a sending probe on the buccal side and a receiving probe on the palatal side of the teeth (figure 2.4). Sasano *et al*, in their experimental study, proved that transmitted laser light assigned all non-vital teeth a zero result, and no interference was evident due to the heart rate creating oscillations in the signal. In additional, when assessing vital teeth, transmitted laser light yielded twice the amplitude of laser Doppler flowmetry, and passive changes in the blood flow were more evident [39, 40].

2.2.1.6 Surface temperature

A balance between the heat brought up to the tooth surface and its dissipation into the surroundings determines the surface temperature of a tooth. In highly controlled surroundings, heat is conducted from the periodontal structure via the roots through the dentin and enamel up to the surface of the tooth. The heat is then carried into the pulp by the circulation. The pulpal metabolism also produces heat in the pulp chamber, which is generally lacking in non-vital teeth. Hence, a temperature difference between heat conduction and pulpal circulation and metabolism can differentiate vital teeth from non-vital teeth. However, this technique has many limitations, such as interference caused by the patient's normal respiration, a long working time, the sensitivity of the technique, and the need for thermally controlled, insulated, draft-free rooms with a temperature maintained at 20° ± 10°C. Fanibunda [41], in an *in vitro* model, connected two thermistors back-to-back; one was in contact with the enamel surface, and the other was suspended in the air. The measuring thermistor in contact with the enamel recorded the crown surface

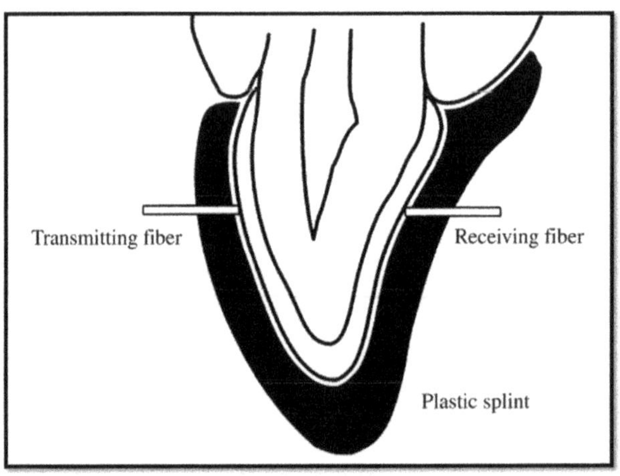

Figure 2.4. A schematic drawing of the transmitted laser light system for monitoring pulpal blood flow [40] John Wiley & Sons. (License No. 5485360301492).

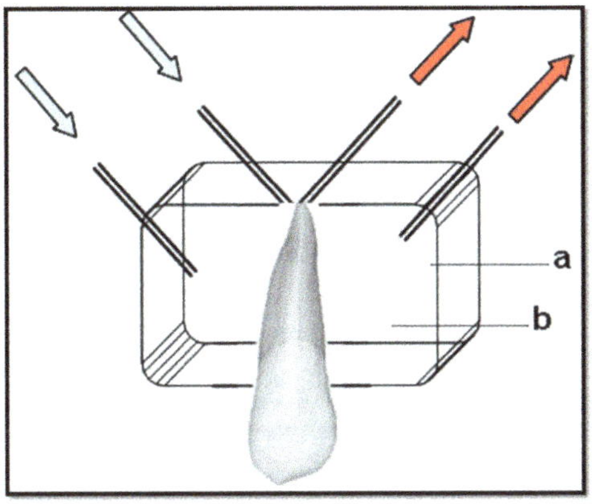

Figure 2.5. A schematic figure for temperature measurement *in vitro* (a, acrylic pouch; b, air space, intended for circulation in the supporting tissue region). The inlet and outlet pipes which are present at the top corner of the pouch are intended to supply the circulating fluid to the supporting tissue. The circulating fluid enters the air space through one pipe and then exits through the other pipe. Reprinted from [45], Copyright (2008), with permission from Elsevier and the American Association of Endodontists.

temperature and the atmospheric temperature, while the reference thermistor measured the atmospheric temperature only. After gaining access to the apical foramen and extirpating the pulp, two tubes serving as an inlet and an outlet were passed through the foramen encased in acrylic; these were particularly aimed at circulating fluid in the supporting tissue (figure 2.5). Although there are various temperature-measuring devices, such as infrared and miniature thermometers, thermistors, and infrared thermography, a few authors have stated that there is no difference between vital and non-vital pulpal temperatures [41–45].

2.2.2 Pulp sensibility

2.2.2.1 Electric pulp test

Electric pulp testing passes an electrical stimulus through the tip of the device through a conducting medium, such as toothpaste, along the prisms and tubules of enamel and dentin, respectively, to the pulp tissue, thereby causing ionic changes in the nerve membrane and inducing an action potential at the nodes of Ranvier of the A-delta fibers [46, 47]. This electrical circuit is usually completed by a lip clip placed on the patient's lip or by holding the probe's handle. The operator can also touch the patient's skin with his gloveless hand as a substitute [48, 49] (figure 2.6). As the voltage increases, the patient usually feels a tingling sensation [50]. However, there is a variation in pain thresholds that depends on the patient and the type of tooth; it is influenced by the patient's age, conduction by the tooth's surface, pain perception, and resistance [47]. There are monopolar and bipolar modes of pulp testers, which can be further categorized into those connected to mains (utility) power and those with batteries. Recent pulp testers are monopolar; the lip clip is considered to be the anode, and the probe tip placed on the tooth is the cathode [51–53].

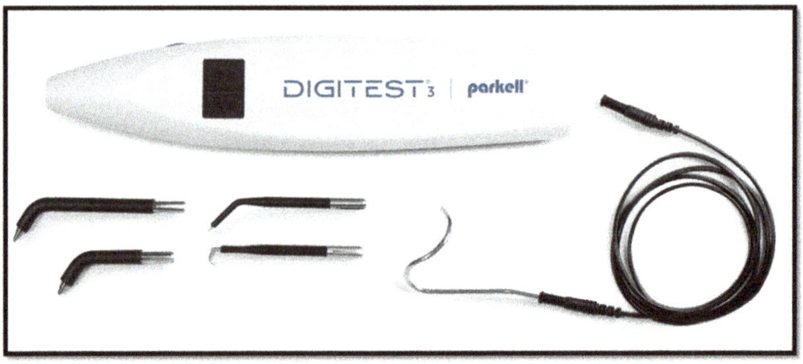

Figure 2.6. Electric Pulp Tester. Courtesy of Parkell Inc.

The pulp tester, however, fails to differentiate between reversible and irreversible pulpitis, as it cannot predict the degree of inflammation [54]. In addition, necrotic teeth with liquid contents can produce false positive reactions [55], and teeth with pulpal calcifications and obliterations, immature teeth, traumatized teeth, those undergoing orthodontic treatment, and patients with primary hyperthyroidism produce false negative reactions from healthy pulps as the sensory responses are either blocked, or more milliamperes of current are required to elicit a reaction [56]. Previous animal studies [57] have shown that pulp testers can interfere with pacemakers; however, due to advancements in medical science, pacemakers with better shielding are not affected by the pulp testers [58–60].

2.3 Caries detection

2.3.1 Fiber-optic transillumination and digital fiber-optic transillumination

Carious tooth structures are more porous than healthy enamel and dentin and absorb and scatter more light photons, thereby appearing darker under trans-illumination, with surrounding tissues appearing white and opaque. FOTI uses optical fibers in a handheld device to transilluminate the tooth structures in the interproximal areas in order to detect incipient carious lesions [61, 62]. DIFOTI is an advancement of FOTI that uses an incorporated handpiece, control panel, image recording system, detection software, and a pedal (figure 2.7). DIFOTI has the advantage of providing *in vivo* digital images with different projection settings for occlusal and interproximal surfaces [63]. *In vitro* [64] and *in vivo* studies [65] have shown that when DIFOTI is compared with radiographic techniques for the detection of interproximal enamel and dentin caries, the accuracy of DIFOTI is greater than the latter for detecting enamel caries, thought it is similar for the detection of dentinal caries (figures 2.8–2.10). A recent Cochrane meta-analysis stated that although FOTI and NILT are readily available and successfully identify good teeth, they have limitations in detecting enamel caries [66].

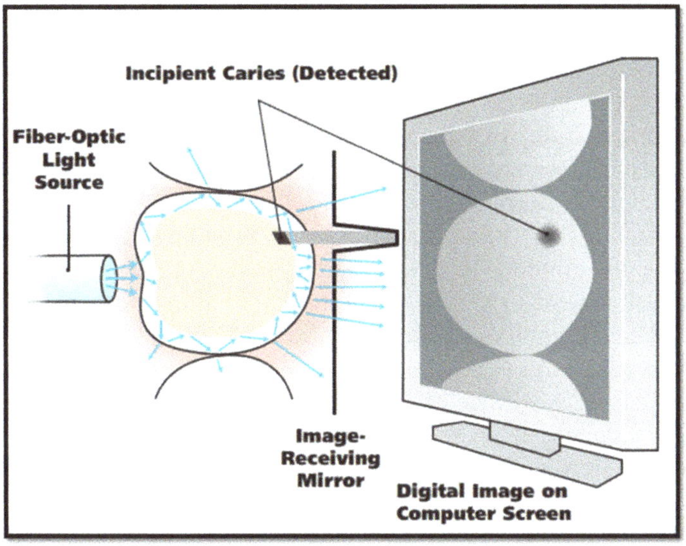

Figure 2.7. The working principle of digital fiber-optic transillumination. Reprinted from [67], Copyright (2008), with permission from Elsevier.

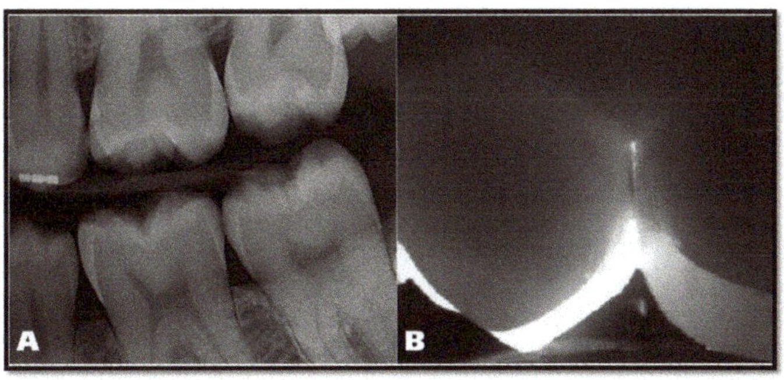

Figure 2.8. Images of a lesion that was scored as 'small.' The lesion is on the distal aspect of the maxillary left second premolar. A. Radiographic image. B. Digital fiber-optic transillumination image. Reprinted from [67], Copyright (2008), with permission from Elsevier.

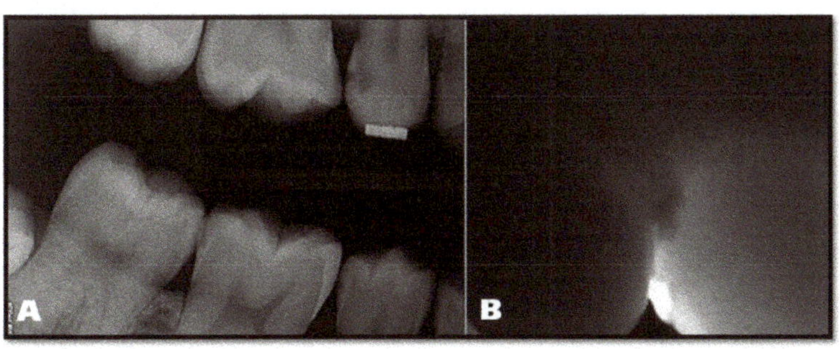

Figure 2.9. Images of a lesion that was scored as 'medium.' The lesion is on the distal aspect of the maxillary right second premolar. A. Radiographic image. B. Digital fiber-optic transillumination image. Reprinted from [67], Copyright (2008), with permission from Elsevier. (License No. 548301144277).

2.3.2 Near-infrared light transillumination

In 2012, Kavo® commercially produced DiagnoCam®, an advanced version of DIFOTI [68]. The device consists of elastic arms containing optical fibers transmitting near-infrared light, a USB connection to a computer, software, and a camera system. The elastic arms are placed near the alveolar process against the tooth's roots, and the light scatters from the occlusal surface, which is captured by the sensor and displayed on the computer by the software. Carious lesions appear darker than the surrounding healthy tissues [69–71]. This device is also based on transillumination, in which visible near-infrared light alternates between 700 nm and 1500 nm [72]. The advantage this method has over DIFOTI is that infrared light at 780 nm disperses less and penetrates deeper, enabling better transmission of light and aiding in incipient caries detection [73]. NILT also differentiates demineralization from other enamel defects such as developmental anomalies, fissures, calculus, pigmentation, or fluorosis [74] (figures 2.11 and 2.12). It also has the advantage of

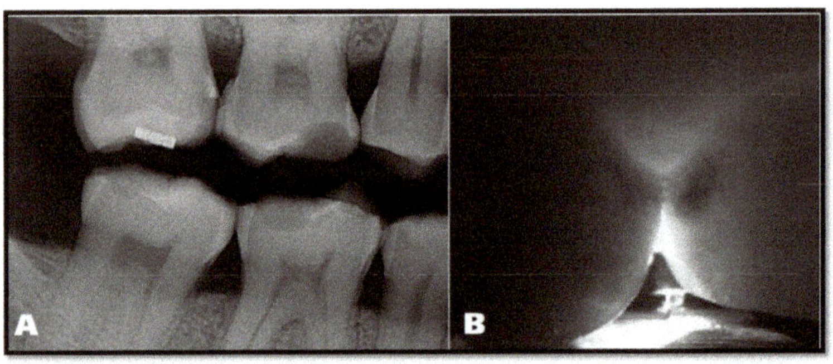

Figure 2.10. Images of lesions that were scored as 'large.' The lesions are on the distal aspect of the maxillary right first molar and the mesial aspect of the maxillary right second molar. A. Radiographic image. B. Digital fiber-optic transillumination image. Reprinted from [67], Copyright (2008), with permission from Elsevier. (License No. 548301144277).

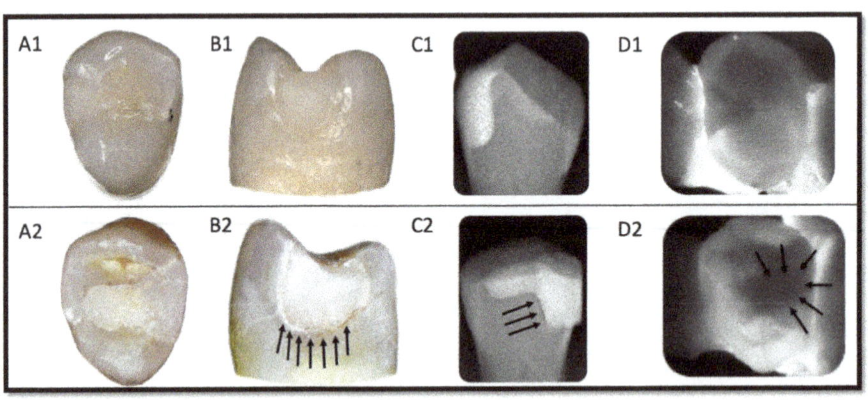

Figure 2.11. Clinical (A; occlusal, B; occlusal proximal view), radiographic (C) and NILT (D) images of teeth. Black arrows indicate the presence of proximal carious lesions adjacent to restorations. Reprinted from [76], Copyright (2018), with permission from Elsevier.

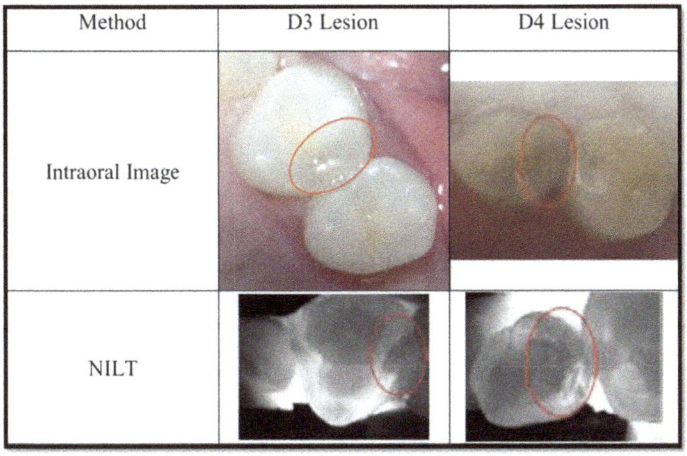

Figure 2.12. A comparison of intraoral and NILT images of teeth [77] (2019). Open access article under CC BY-SA. With permission of Springer.

being nonionizing, aiding the clinician in diagnosing a quadrant within half a minute, as one image per surface is created within 40 milliseconds. However, the limitations of the device include its inability to detect subgingival caries, periodontal structures, and caries under large restorations and crowns [75].

2.3.3 Optical coherence tomography

Optical coherence tomography is a nonionizing, noninvasive technique based on interferometry. It uses a beam of partially coherent light consisting of near-infrared light waves to create tomographic images by reflecting from microstructures. Real-time images are obtained with an exceptional axial resolution of less than 10 μm [78]. Time-domain optical coherence tomography (TdOCT) and Fourier-domain optical coherence tomography (FdOCT) are two basic types of OCT. TdOCT was developed in 1991 for ophthalmic diagnosis at the Massachusetts Institute of Technology in the United States [79]. It has a long measurement time, and the resulting images are of poor quality. In addition, it does not allow for 3D imaging. Hence, FdOCT was developed; it has a capture time a hundred times shorter than that of TdOCT and the added advantage of producing 3D images.

The location of scattering along the primary beam is contained in the modulation frequency of the near-infrared light intensity and is measured as a function of frequency. The electric signal produced by the spectral detection of interfering beams is called the signal of spectral bands. Spectral OCT and swept-source OCT (SS-OCT) or optical Fourier-domain imaging (OFDI) are two methods for detecting these signals. The striking difference between the above and TdOCT is the presence of fixed reference mirrors [80] (figure 2.13).

In addition to its use in caries detection, OCT has other applications in dentistry, such as the diagnosis of cracks, soft tissue pathoses, and oral cancer, the detection of root canals, alveolar bone loss, plaques, and nearby anatomical areas, and the

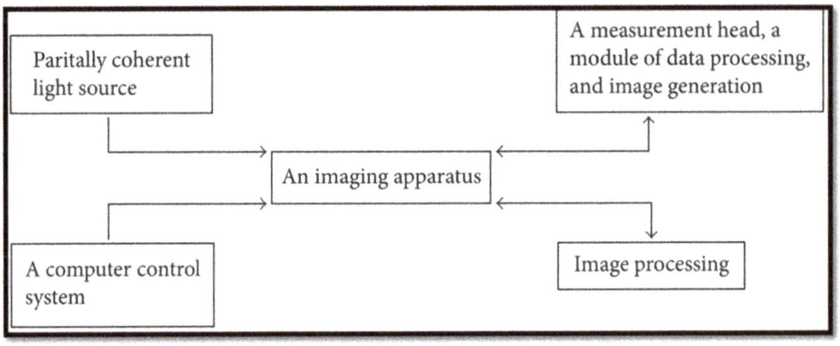

Figure 2.13. The operating principle of optical coherence tomography. Reproduced from [81]. CC BY 4.0. Copyright © 2017 Monika Machoy et al.

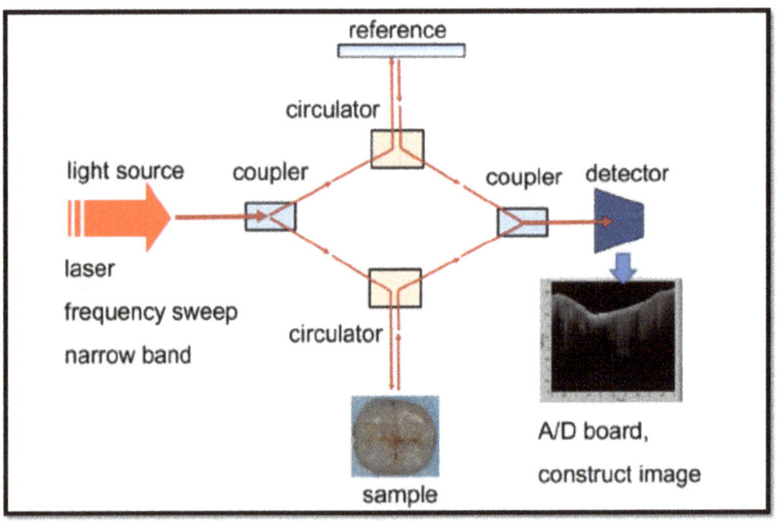

Figure 2.14. A schematic illustration of an SS-OCT system. Reprinted from [83], Copyright (2020), with permission from Elsevier

evaluation of prostheses and restorations [82]. Macey *et al*, in their systematic review, stated that OCT is superior to NILT and FOTI devices for the detection of enamel caries [66].

SS-OCT is a modification of FdOCT that has detectors to measure interference versus time, a narrow-linewidth interferometer, and a frequency-swept laser [83] (figure 2.14). In contrast to the radiographic appearance of dental caries, demineralized lesions appear white in SS-OCT images due to increased backscatter [84, 85].

However, OCT has a few limitations, including a low scanning range of several millimeters, which leads to many pictures of an entire lesion. This can be overcome by developing a dental optical probe that can screen the entire lesion and focus on specific areas. Additionally, its poor penetration depth restricts the usage of OCT in daily clinical practice [81].

2.3.4 Electrical conductance and impedance

In 1878, Magitot first suggested using electrical current to detect dental caries [86]. This use of electrical conductance is based on the principle that sound enamel has low percentages of fluid and porosity and is hence a poor conductor of electricity; however, with the development of dental caries, porosity and fluid increase within the affected areas, thus creating a conducive environment for the passage of electricity [87]. Two commercially available devices based on this principle are the Electronic Caries Monitor® and the CarieScan Pro®. The former is based on electrical conductivity, while the latter is based on impedance [88].

2.3.4.1 The Electronic Caries Monitor®

This device uses a single-, fixed-frequency alternating current to assess the bulk resistance of the tooth [89]. Its electrical conductance is influenced by the porosity, contact area, thickness, and hydration of the enamel, along with the ionic contents of the surrounding fluids [90]. The research literature has proven this method of caries assessment to be superior to FOTI and radiographs for the detection of early lesions. However, stains, variations in reproducibility, and probe contact with the tooth surface represent limitations [91–93].

2.3.4.2 The CarieScan Pro®

This device measures the electrical impedance on a scale that gives information about the severity of dental caries. Impedance measures the degree of resistance of an electrical circuit to current flow when voltage is applied between two electrodes. If a direct current is applied, the impedance corresponds to resistance, whereas in alternating-current circuits, it corresponds to resistance, inductance, and capacitance [94]. The device employs a range of alternating-current frequencies (100 Hz–100 kHz), thereby creating a spectrum of impedance points (10 kΩ–10 MΩ) with a maximum error of 5% [95]. This technique is known as the alternating-current impedance spectroscopy technique. Teeth with dental caries have lower impedance and higher conductivity than healthy tooth structures (figure 2.15).

Similarly, immature enamel and dentin have higher conductivity than mature enamel. The CarieScan Pro® consists of a metallic probe placed on the tooth, a lip hook attached to the patient's lip, and an LED screen that displays numerical values. After the tooth is cleaned and dried, the probe is placed on the surface to be assessing, which results in a score and color ranging from zero to 100; green implies a sound tooth and red implies carious activity. The higher the numerical value, the more advanced the carious lesions are, and hence the lower their electrical impedance [96]. When the score ranges between one and 50, a green–yellow bar code is seen on the screen, corresponding to a low probability of caries; scores of 51–90 correspond to yellow–orange colors, and scores of 91–99 correspond to orange–red colors, representing medium and high probabilities of caries, respectively [97]. The limitations of the device include its inability to monitor cavitated lesions, root caries, and secondary caries; the dentin is exposed in the former, which therefore always has higher electrical conductance and always reads 100; interfering

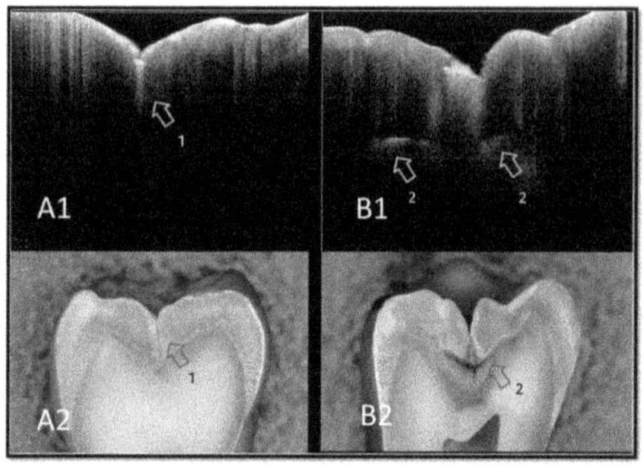

Figure 2.15. Swept-source optical coherence tomography (SS-OCT) images of occlusal caries obtained noninvasively (A1, B1) and the corresponding histological view after cross-sectioning (A2, B2). Enamel demineralization at an occlusal fissure is imaged as increased brightness within the depth of the dentin–enamel junction (DEJ) (arrow 1). The presence of hidden dentin caries is depicted in SS-OCT as a backscattering signal from the lesion boundary (B1). The extent of the lesion along the DEJ is imaged as a bright line (arrow 2). Reprinted from [83], Copyright (2020), with permission from Elsevier

dental materials are present in the latter, which makes it difficult to detect caries around them. The probe can be used only on occlusal and smooth surfaces and is avoided in patients with cardiac pacemakers [88]. A meta-analysis stated that the sensitivities of the Electrical Caries Monitor® and the CarieScan Pro® are 0.61–0.98 and 0.55–0.91, respectively, while their specificities are 0.73–0.96 and 0–1.0, respectively [98].

2.3.5 Fluorescence-based devices and techniques

2.3.5.1 DIAGNOdent®

The DIAGNOdent 2095 and The DIAGNOdent 2190 (KaVo Dental, Lake Zurich, IL, USA) are devices based on laser fluorescence. They emit a monochromatic red laser beam at 655 nm which excites bacterial photo porphyrins, ultimately resulting in detectable fluorescence. The backscattered waves reach the detector, and the signals are modulated and strengthened to give the respective values. As the carious activity increases, the scattering within the tooth microstructure increases, increasing the level of fluorescence [99]. The DIAGNOdent values range from 0–99, wherein 0–12 denotes a healthy state, 13–24 denotes demineralized enamel, and >25 shows the involvement of dentin [88]. The limitations of this device include unreliability in the presence of confounding factors such as stains and restorative materials [100, 101]. The sensitivity of the device is high in comparison to its specificity, as the device requires additional detection aids [102–104].

2.3.5.2 Midwest Caries ID

The Midwest Caries ID (Dentsply, York, PA, USA) analyzes the translucency and opacity of the tooth microstructure by determining the mineral content and integrity of enamel rods based on the reflection and refraction of light emitted by the analyzed surface. It is based on LED technology; its incident light has wavelengths between

635 nm and 880 nm, and the emitted light is captured by fiber optics that convert it into electrical signals for further analysis. When the severity of the lesion increases, the LED changes from green to red with an added audible signal. However, the minimal published literature indicates the device's lack of differentiation of enamel caries from sound tooth structure [105, 106].

2.3.5.3 VistaCam®

The VistaCam® camera (Classic, CL, and IX) (Durr Dental, Germany) is based on intraoral fluorescence. It consists of six violet LEDs that generate light at a wavelength of 405 nm. The camera, when shone on a tooth surface, illuminates the tooth and captures the reflected light, which is filtered for light below 495 nm to differentiate healthy teeth from carious lesions. The former emit a green/yellow fluorescence which peaks at 510 nm and the latter emit a red fluorescence that peaks at 680 nm. The red and green fluorescences are then quantified as numerical values ranging from zero to three. These depict the severity and advancement of the carious lesion based on the DBSWIN software program provided with the device [107–109]. The respective codes have the following meanings: 0–1—healthy enamel,1–1.5—initial enamel demineralization, 1.5–2—deep enamel decay, 2–2.5—dentin caries, and 2.5–3—deep dentin caries [88] (figure 2.16).

2.3.5.4 The Soprolife® system

The Soprolife® device (Acteon, La Ciotat, France) is equipped with an intraoral camera that consists of two types of LED which illuminate either in the white light region or in a narrow band at a wavelength of 450 nm and a bandwidth of 20 nm.

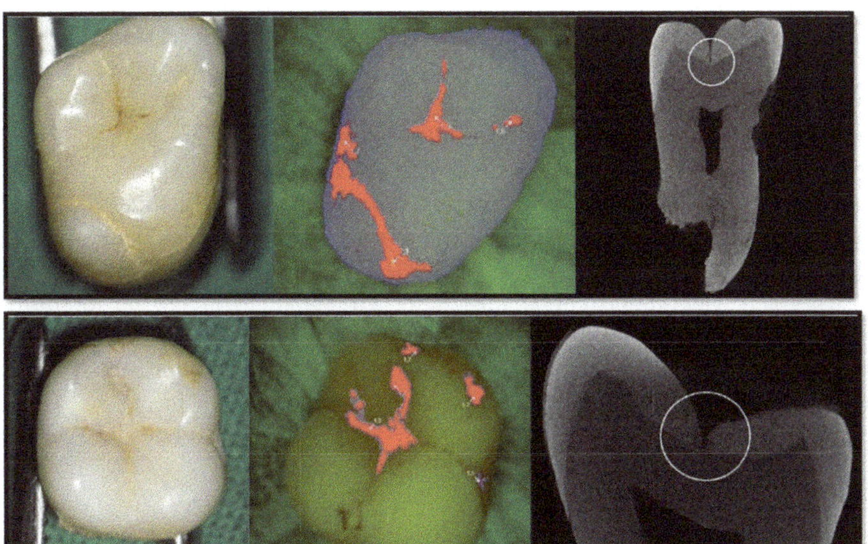

Figure 2.16. Discoloration in the fissures (left picture) on the upper second molar and lower second molar, VistaCam image (central picture) and initial caries as confirmed by micro-CT (right picture) [110] John Wiley & Sons. © 2014 Wiley Periodicals, Inc.

The device is equipped to diagnose and detect any local differences in density, composition, and structure by providing an anatomical image that is superimposed on an autofluorescence image. The device illuminates in one frequency band, and the resultant fluorescence occurs in a second band which is picked up by a camera consisting of 0.25 inch CCD sensors with a mosaic of pixels that allows the retrieval of an image. The camera operates with four white LEDs in its daylight mode, whereas four blue LEDs are illuminated for its diagnostic and treatment modes. Soprocare®, a new camera addition, works in three modes: daylight, caries, and periodontal, focusing on inflammatory changes in the periodontium. The camera is based on the light-induced fluorescence evaluator for diagnosis and treatment (LIFEDT) concept, whose principles include

- cleaning of the assessed tooth surface areas,
- observation at high magnification in the daylight and fluorescent modes, and
- analyzing the reflected light in comparison to healthy areas.

The Soproimaging® software records and compares the obtained pictures [111, 112]. Scoring in the blue fluorescent mode is shown in figure 2.17.

2.3.5.5 SiroInspect

SiroInspect® (Dentsply Sirona, Germany) illuminates the tooth with violet light at a wavelength of 405 nm, stimulating the decomposition products of the carious dentin, including the healthy tooth structure (figure 2.18). The filter removes the light of shorter wavelengths below 500 nm; hence, the carious tissue fluoresces red, whereas healthy tissue is green. The device incorporates Fluorescence-Aided Caries Excavation (FACE), with which a clinician with special glasses can visualize the fluorescence in the tooth and further provide a therapeutic measure to remove and reconstruct the remineralized areas. However, these systems do not record images [114, 115].

2.4.5.6 Quantitative light- (or laser-) induced fluorescence

Quantitative light- (or laser-) induced fluorescence (QLF), an intraoral imaging technique, is based on the property of fluorescence, which is the emission of light at higher wavelengths following the absorption of incident light at a shorter wavelength (figure 2.19). As the carious activity progresses into the dentin, the incident light scatters more; hence, the fluorescence is reduced [116]. The demineralized area appears dark against a green background [90] (figure 2.20). The captured image can quantify the amount of lost fluorescence and surface area using software; it can also be superimposed on successive images to detect the carious lesion's remineralization post-therapeutic interventions visually. Although QLF can identify precavitated or incipient lesions, it is expensive and technique sensitive and can only be used on accessible surfaces [117].

2.3.5.7 Photothermal radiometry and modulated luminescence

Mandelis *et al* [120] and Nicolaides *et al* [121] first reported the diagnostic capability of noninvasive frequency-domain photothermal radiometry to detect dental defects. When this was an adjunct to modulated luminescence, early detection of dental caries was possible [122, 123]. Photothermal radiometry and modulated

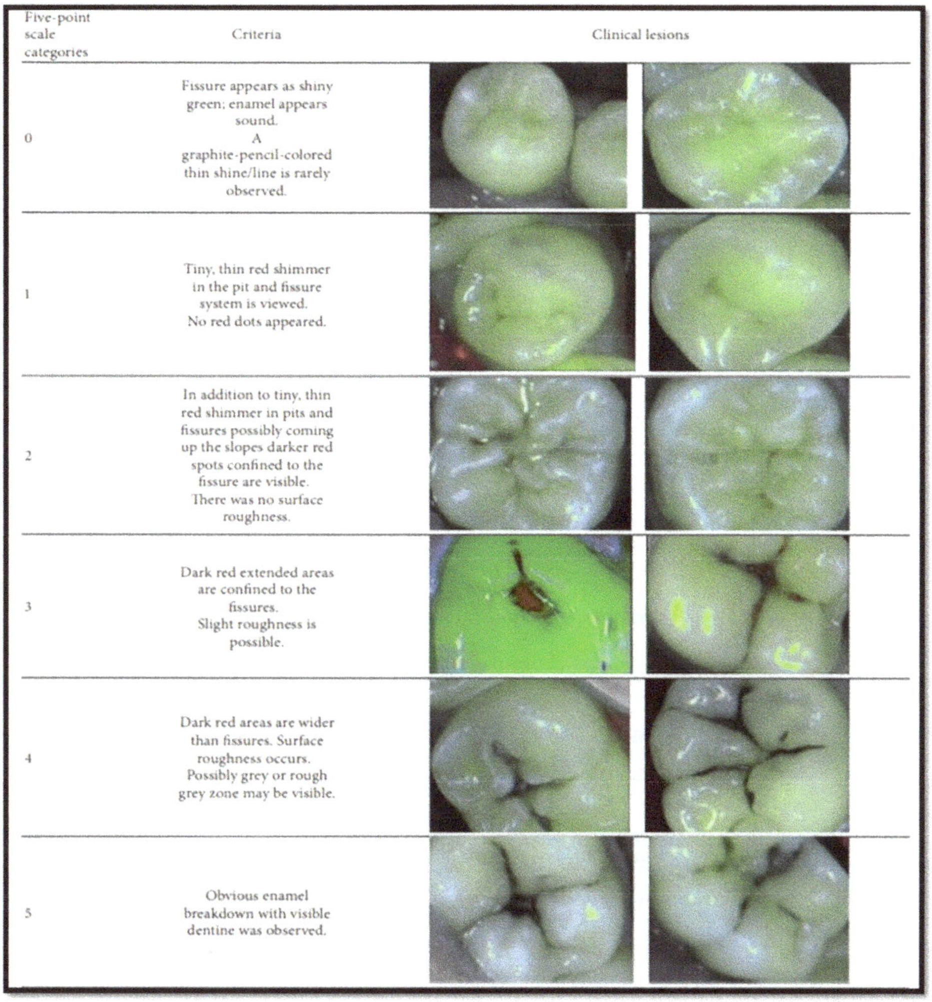

Five-point scale categories	Criteria	Clinical lesions
0	Fissure appears as shiny green; enamel appears sound. A graphite-pencil-colored thin shine/line is rarely observed.	
1	Tiny, thin red shimmer in the pit and fissure system is viewed. No red dots appeared.	
2	In addition to tiny, thin red shimmer in pits and fissures possibly coming up the slopes darker red spots confined to the fissure are visible. There was no surface roughness.	
3	Dark red extended areas are confined to the fissures. Slight roughness is possible.	
4	Dark red areas are wider than fissures. Surface roughness occurs. Possibly grey or rough grey zone may be visible.	
5	Obvious enamel breakdown with visible dentine was observed.	

Figure 2.17. Soprolife scores in the blue fluorescence mode. Reproduced from [113]. CC BY 4.0. Copyright © 2014 Mona Zeitouny et al.

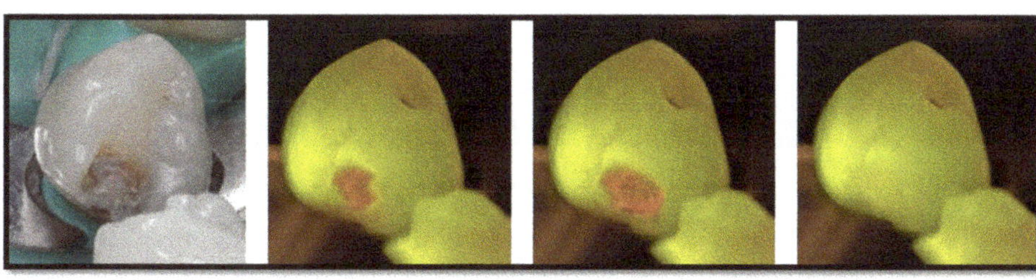

Figure 2.18. SiroInspect. ©2016 DENTSPLY SIRON.

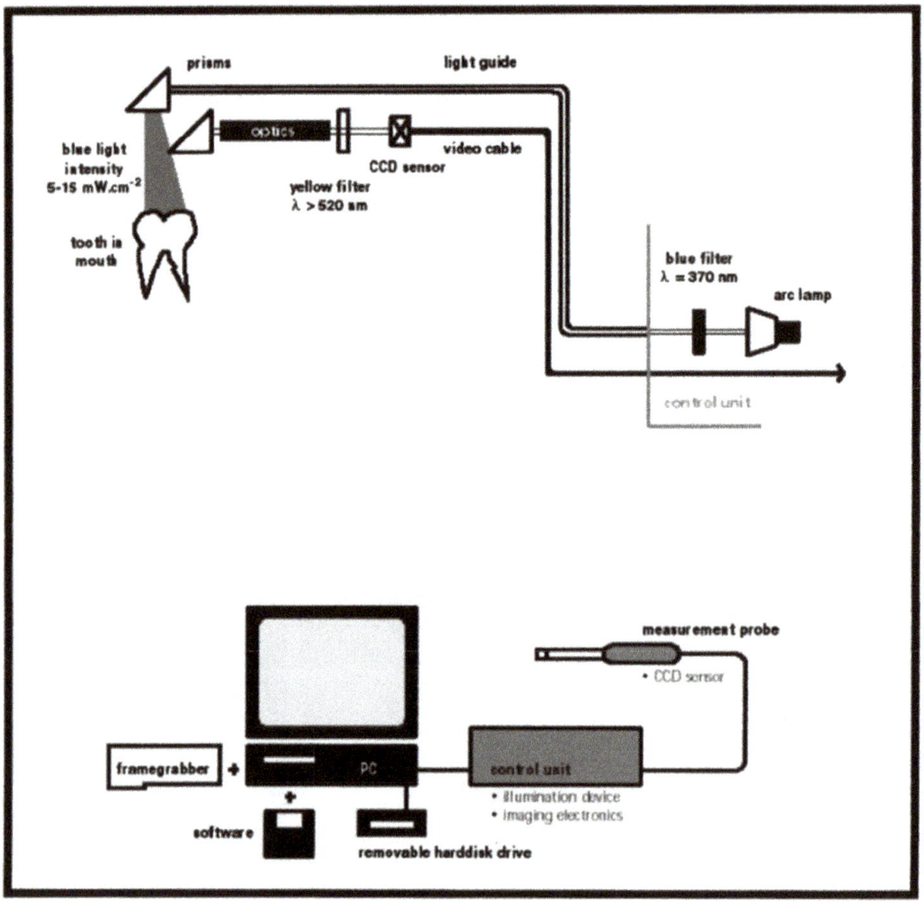

Figure 2.19. A schematic illustration of the quantitative light- (or laser-) induced fluorescence clinical system. Reprinted from [118] ©(2002) Society of Photo-Optical Instrumentation Engineers (SPIE)

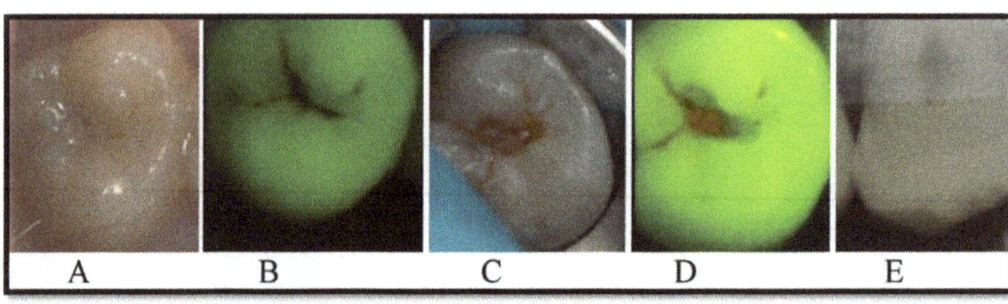

Figure 2.20. (A) A white light image of a molar with a suspected carious area, (B) a QLF image showing demineralized areas, (C) a white light image after initial preparation confirming the presence of caries, (D) a QLF image of a tooth showing localized areas of decay (dark spots) and red fluorescence and (E) a radiograph showing no evidence of caries. Reprinted from [119], Copyright (2013), with permission from Elsevier.

luminescence (PTR-LUM) consists of modulated thermal infrared radiation and alternating-current luminescence [124].

When laser light is modulated at a specific frequency and incident on a tooth, radiation of a similar frequency is emitted by the tooth along with the radiative conversion of optical energy to longer wavelengths, heat released in the form of thermal infrared photons of the same frequency, and finally non-radiative conversion of the remaining energy. Hence, the converted heat and light energy from the incident laser beam, along with the intensity modulation and time delay due to heat conduction, are measured by PTR-LUM. Unlike optical energy, PTR-LUM does not scatter. With the advancement of carious activity/demineralization, the amount of infrared radiation and luminescence collected is equivalent to the incident energy, and the exact opposite occurs with remineralization. Hence, photonic devices employing PTR-LUM can aid in detecting and diagnosing small carious lesions [125, 126].

The Canary System® is a noninvasive energy conversion system employing PTR-LUM, which assesses the tooth microstructure based on combined optical and thermal data. Low-power lasers pulsating at a frequency of 2 Hz are shone on the tooth for a 3 s duration, generating PTR-LUM responses and detecting caries with an intraoral camera [127]. The Canary System has a probing area and a depth of 1.5 mm and up to 5 mm, respectively and can detect carious lesions as small as 50 microns. The number displayed can range from zero to 100; scores of 0–20 signify healthy teeth, 21–70 signify decay, and 71–100 signify an advanced carious lesion [128].

In summary, fluorescence-based devices can be categorized into red, green, and blue fluorescence-emitting devices. The red fluorescence devices use a small laser with an excitation wavelength greater than 655 nm; examples include the DIAGNOdent and DIAGNOdent pen, MidWest, and the Canary System. Blue fluorescence devices work at wavelengths ranging between 400 and 450 nm in the violet light spectrum, in which carious teeth create luminescence and healthy teeth fluoresce green. The devices falling into this category are the Vistaproof, SoproLife, and Spectra. QLF is an example of a green fluorescence device that relies on the green–yellow spectrum at a wavelength of 370 nm [129]. A meta-analysis has stated that all the fluorescence-based devices have similar performance but better accuracy in detecting advanced lesions [130].

2.4 Root canal length determination

2.4.1 The electronic apex locator (EAL)

According to the glossary of endodontic terms, the working length is defined as ‘the distance from a coronal reference point to the point at which canal preparation and obturation should terminate,’ and an apex locator is ‘an electronic instrument used to assist in determining the root canal working length or perforation; operates on the principles of resistance, frequency or impedance.’

Apex locators work by completing an electrical circuit, one side of which is attached to the patient’s lip, contacting the oral mucosa, and the other side of which is attached to a file placed inside the root canal. The basic principle is that the electrical resistance between the mucous membrane and periodontal structures is

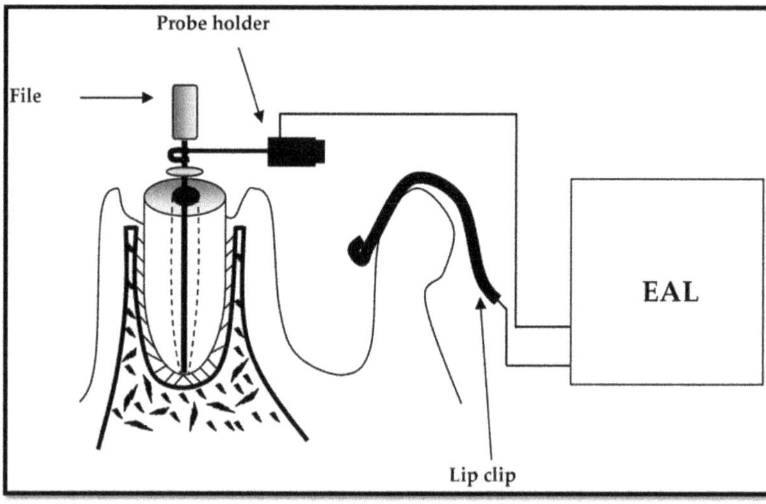

Figure 2.21. The mechanism of the electronic apex locator. Reprinted from [132]. Courtesy of Tokyo Medical and Dental University Library © 2007 Tokyo Medical and Dental University (TMDU).

6 kΩ in any part of the periodontium, irrespective of age, shape, and type of tooth. With the advancement of the file into the canal towards the root apex, when the circuit is completed and the resistance between the file and mucosa is equal, a signal is visualized, confirming that the file is at the apex [131, 132] (figure 2.21). Four generations of apex locators have worked on alternating current based on resistance, impedance, and frequency (the subtraction and ratio types) [133].

2.4.2 Periapical lesion detection and differentiation

2.4.2.1 Magnetic resonance imaging

MRI is a nonionizing, noninvasive diagnostic tool that aids in understanding root canal anatomy, periapical lesion detection and differentiation, the detection of caries, cracks, pulp vitality, and pulp regeneration/reperfusion, assessments of stem-cell-based regeneration, and endodontic treatment prediction.

MRI visualizes periapical granuloma as an ill-defined outer margin with involvement in the surrounding soft tissue and a wide peripheral rim with an inhomogeneous texture at the lesion center. In contrast, a cyst appears as a well-defined outer margin without soft tissue involvement and a thin peripheral rim with a homogeneous texture at the lesion center [134].

The working mechanism of MRI depends on the hydrogen protons present in every living tissue. The hydrogen protons spin about their axes, and when the patient is placed in a magnetic field, the nuclei align to the direction of the magnetic field. When a radio-frequency wave is sent, it affects all the hydrogen protons and alters their movement from the longitudinal to the transverse plane. On stoppage of the radio-frequency signal, the nuclei lose energy and return to their equilibratory longitudinal axis, producing a measurable signal. This process is called relaxation [135, 136].

2.4.2.2 Ultrasound

Ultrasound is a nonionizing, noninvasive, and real-time imaging method based on sound waves' reflection and echo. It employs a transducer that transmits high-frequency pulses in the range of 1–20 MHz. The waves on returning to the transducer differ in gray scale based on the density of the tissues [137]. In dentistry, ultrasound has just entered the array of available diagnostic modalities and aids in diagnosing and differentiating periapical lesions, determining pulp vitality, detecting caries and cracks, and sinus tracing.

In an ultrasound image, a periapical cyst is visualized as a hypoechoic, well-contoured cavity surrounded by reinforced bone walls and filled with fluid; it shows no evidence of internal vasculature on color and power Doppler examinations. In contrast, granuloma appears as a poorly defined lesion, which can be hyperechoic/echogenic or have both hyperechoic and hypoechoic areas and exhibits a rich vascular supply on color and power Doppler examinations [138] (figure 2.22). A recent systematic review also states that the sensitivity and specificity of ultrasound

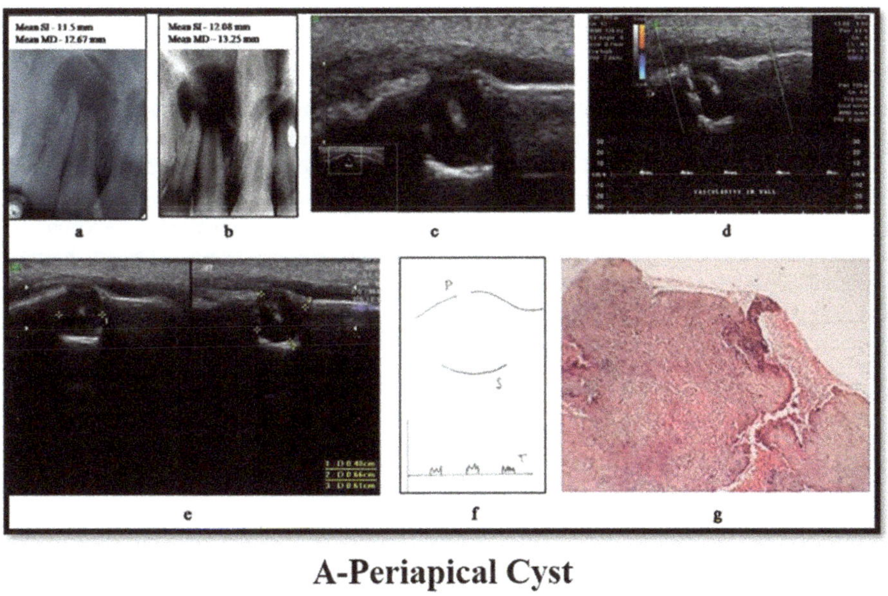

Figure 2.22A. A case of a periapical cyst. (a) A conventional radiograph, and (b) a digital image, showing well-defined periapical radiolucency with sclerotic borders in relation to the right maxillary central and lateral incisors; it includes superoinferior and mesiodistal measurements of a lesion. (c) As ultrasound image shown on a monitor in split-screen mode shows the surface of a thinned buccal cortical plate of bone (P), the deep surface (S) of a periapical lesion, and an anechoic area in between P and S due to fluid content. (d) No evidence of vascularization in the wall on color Doppler examination. (e) An ultrasound image showing superoinferior, mesiodistal, and anteroposterior measurements of a lesion. (f) The diagrammatic equivalents of (c) and (d). (e) A histopathologic picture, showing a cystic epithelium 6–8 cell layers thick proliferating into the stroma in an arcading pattern, underlying connective tissue with loosely arranged collagen fibers, mild to moderate inflammatory cell infiltration, and numerous endothelium-lined blood vessels and extravasated red blood cells. Reprinted from [140], Copyright (2010), with permission from Elsevier. © 2010 Mosby, Inc. Published by Elsevier Inc. All rights reserved.

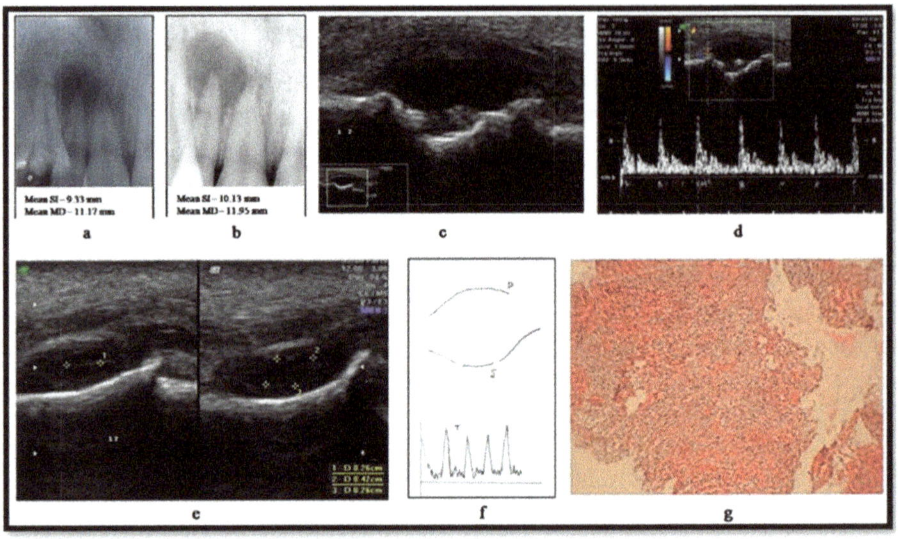

B-Periapical Granuloma

Figure 2.22B. A case of periapical granuloma. (a) A conventional radiograph, and (b) a digital image showing well circumscribed periapical radiolucency in relation to the right maxillary central and lateral incisors and superoinferior and mesiodistal measurements of a lesion. (c) An ultrasound image shown on a monitor in split-screen mode shows surface of a thinned buccal cortical plate of bone (P), the deep surface (S) of a periapical lesion, and a hypoechoic area in between P and S. (d) A spectral Doppler T trace showing blood flow. (e) An ultrasound image showing superoinferior, mesiodistal, and anteroposterior measurements of a lesion. (f) The diagrammatic equivalent of (c) and (d). (e) A histopathologic picture, showing connective tissue with immature to mature collagen fibers arranged in bundles and diffuse mild to moderate chronic inflammatory cell infiltration with hemorrhagic areas; no lining epithelium was evident. Reprinted from [140], Copyright (2010), with permission from Elsevier.© 2010 Mosby, Inc. Published by Elsevier Inc. All rights reserved.

in diagnosing periapical cysts and periapical granulomas were high and that these methods were accurate and almost similar to histopathology, which is advantageous, as the former is noninvasive [139].

2.5 Conclusions

As a result of advancements in diagnostic modalities in endodontics, the role of harmful radiation is seemingly decreasing. These technologies are now readily available to clinicians, which aids in data collection, treatment planning, and, finally, performing minimally invasive endodontic procedures with the help of the information obtained. As the world of dentistry moves towards the conservation of the natural tooth structure, the introduction of these noninvasive, nonionizing diagnostics seems to be a boon. The importance of pulp vitality testing, early carious lesion detection, tooth apex location, and periapical lesion detection and differentiation in endodontics have led to the evolution of these novel diagnostic modalities.

Conflicts of interest

Nil

Sources of funding

Nil

References

[1] Persoon I F and Ozok A R 2017 Definitions and epidemiology of Endodontic infections *Curr. Oral Health Rep.* **4** 278–85
[2] Morgan W F and Bair W J 2012 Issues in low dose radiation biology: the controversy continues. A perspective *Radiat. Res.* **179** 501–10
[3] Tapp J V and Kron T (ed) 2008 *An Introduction to Radiation Protection in Medicine* (Boca Raton, FL: CRC Press)
[4] McMorrow R C and Mythen M G 2006 Pulse oximetry *Curr. Opin. Crit. Care* **12** 269–71
[5] American Medical Association 1993 The use of pulse oximetry during conscious sedation. Council on scientific affairs, american medical association *J. Am. Dent. Assoc.* **270** 1463–8
[6] Schnapp L M and Cohen N H 1990 Pulse oximetry: uses and abuses *Chest* **98** 244–50
[7] Benaron D A, Benitz W E, Ariagnos R L and Stevenson D K 1992 Noninvasive methods for estimating *in vivo* oxygenation *Clin. Pediatr.* **31** 258–73
[8] Coble Y D Jr, Eisenbrey A B and Estes E H Jr 1993 The use of pulse oximetry during conscious sedation *JAMA* **270** 1463–8
[9] Bowes W A, Corke B C and Hulka J 1989 Pulse oximetry: a review of the theory, accuracy, and clinical applications *Obstet. Gynecol.* **74** 541–6 https://journals.lww.com/greenjournal/Abstract/1989/09002/PULSE_OXIMETRY__A_REVIEW_OF_THE_THEORY,_ACCURACY,.35.aspx
[10] Mendelson Y 1992 Pulse oximetry: theory and applications for noninvasive monitoring *Clin. Chem.* **38** 601–7
[11] McGough E K and Boysen P G 1989 Benefits and limitations of pulse oximetry in the I.C.U. *J. Crit. Ill.* **4** 23–31
[12] Mardirossian G and Schneider R E 1992 Limitations of pulse oximetry *Anesth. Prog.* **39** 194–6
[13] Gopikrishna V, Tinagupta K and Kandaswamy D 2007 Evaluation of efficacy of a new custom-made pulse oximeter dental probe in comparison with the electrical and thermal tests for assessing pulp vitality *J. Endod.* **33** 411–4
[14] Patro S *et al* 2022 Diagnostic accuracy of pulp vitality tests and pulp sensibility tests for assessing pulpal health in permanent teeth: a systematic review and meta-analysis *Int. J. Environ. Res. Public Health* **19** 9599
[15] Mainkar A and Kim S G 2018 Diagnostic accuracy of 5 dental pulp tests: a systematic review and meta-analysis *J. Endod.* **44** 694–702
[16] Dastmalchi N, Jafarzadeh H and Moradi S 2012 Comparison of the efficacy of a custom-made pulse oximeter probe with digital electric pulp tester, cold spray, and rubber cup for assessing pulp vitality *J. Endod.* **38** 1182–6
[17] Kahan R S, Gulabivala K, Snook M and Setchell D J. 1996 Evaluation of a pulse oximeter and customized probe for pulp vitality testing *J. Endod.* **22** 105–9

[18] Bruno K, Brando Barletta F, Tadeau Felippe W, Almeida Silva J, Gonçalves de Alencar A H and Estrela C 2014 Oxygen saturation in the dental pulp of permanent teeth: a critical review *J. Endod.* **40** 1054–7

[19] Pozzobon M H, Sousa Vieira R, Hecke Alves A M, Reyes-Carmona J, Silveira Teixeira C, Mendes de Souza B C and Tadeu Felippe W 2011 Assessment of pulp blood flow in primary and permanent teeth using pulse oximetry *Dent. Traumatol.* **27** 184–8

[20] Riva C E 2001 Basic principles of laser Doppler flowmetry and application to the ocular circulation *Int. Ophthalmol.* **23** 183–9

[21] Kimura Y, Wilder-Smith P and Matsumoto K 2000 Lasers in Endodontics: a review *Int. Endodontic J.* **33** 173–85

[22] Gazelius B, Olgart L, Edwall B and Edwall L 1986 Non-invasive recording of blood flow in human dental pulp *Endod. Dent. Traumatol.* **2** 219–21

[23] Bonner R F and Nossal R 1990 Principles of laser-Doppler flowmetry *Laser-Doppler Blood Flowmetry* ed A P Shepherd and P A Oberg (New York: Springer) 390–409

[24] Rowe A H R and Pitt Ford T R 1990 The assessment of pulpal vitality *Int. Endodontic J.* **23** 77–83

[25] Roeykens H J J, Van Maele G O G, De Moor R J C and Martens L C M 1999 Reliability of laser Doppler flowmetry in a 2-probe assessment of pulpal blood flow *Oral Surg. Oral Med. Oral Pathol. Oral Radiol. Endod.* **87** 742–8

[26] Albrecht H E, Damaschke N, Borys M and Tropea C 2003 *Laser Doppler and Phase Doppler Measurement Techniques* (New York: Springer) 4–30 pp

[27] Jafarzadeh H 2009 Laser Doppler flowmetry in endodontics: a review *Int. Endod. J.* **42** 476–90

[28] Berman L H and Hartwell G R 2006 Diagnosis *Pathways of the Pulp* ed S Cohen and K M Hargreaves 9th edn (St. Louis, MO: Mosby) 1 16–20

[29] Roebuck E M, Evans D J P, Stirrups D and Strang R 2000 The effect of wavelength, bandwidth, and probe design and position on assessing the vitality of anterior teeth with laser Doppler flowmetry *Int. J. Paediatr. Dent.* **10** 213–20

[30] Matthews B and Vongsavan N 1993 Advantages and limitations of laser Doppler flow meters *Int. Endodontic J.* **26** 9–10

[31] Edwall B, Gazelius B, Berg J-O, Edwall L, Hellander K and Olgart L 1987 Blood flow changes in the dental pulp of the cat and rat measured simultaneously by laser Doppler flowmetry and local 125I clearance *Acta Physiol. Scand.* **131** 81–91

[32] Schmitt J M, Webber R L and Walker E C 1991 Optical determination of dental pulp vitality *IEEE Trans. Biomed. Eng.* **38** 346–52

[33] Shoher Y, Mahler and Samueloff S 1973 Dental pulp photoplethysmography in human beings *Oral Surg. Oral Med. Oral Pathol.* **36** 915–21

[34] Chen E and Abbott P V 2009 Dental pulp testing: a review *Int. J. Dent.* **12** 365785

[35] Knörzer S, Hiller K A, Brandt M, Niklas A, Putzger J, Monkman G J, Danilov S N, Ganichev S D, Schulz I and Schmalz G 2019 Detection of pulsed blood flow through a molar pulp chamber and surrounding tissue *in vitro Clin. Oral Investig.* **23** 1121–32

[36] Miwa Z, Ikawa M, Iijima H, Saito M and Takagi Y 2002 Pulpal blood flow in vital and nonvital young permanent teeth measured by transmitted-light photoplethysmography: a pilot study *Pediatr. Dent.* **24** 594–8

[37] Nivesh P S 2016 Recent diagnostic aids in endodontics—a review *Int. J. Pharm. Chem. Res.* **8** 1159–62

[38] Nissan R, Trope M, Zhang C-D and Chance B 1992 Dual wavelength Spectrophotometry as a diagnostic test of the pulp chamber contents *Oral Surg. Oral Med. Oral Pathol.* **74** 508–14
[39] Sasano T, Nakajima I and Shoji N 1997 Possible application of transmitted laser light I for the assessment of human pulpal vitality *Endod. Dent. Traumatol.* **13** 88–91
[40] Sasano T, Onodera D and Hashimoto K *et al* 2005 Possible application of transmitted laser light for the assessment of human pulp vitality—part 2: increased laser power for enhanced detection of pulpal blood flow *Dent. Traumatol.* **21** 37–41
[41] Fanibunda K B 1986 The feasibility of temperature measurement as a diagnostic procedure in human teeth *J. Dentistry* **14** 126–9
[42] Banes J D and Hammond H L 1978 Surface temperatures of vital and nonvital teeth in humans *J. Endodontics* **4** 106–9
[43] Stoops L C and Scott D Jr 1976 Measurement of tooth temperature as a means of determining pulp vitality *J. Endodontics* **2** 141–5
[44] Brown A C and Goldberg M P 1966 Surface temperature and temperature gradients of human teeth *in situ Arch. Oral Biol.* **11** 973–82
[45] Jafarzadeh H, Udoye C I and Kinoshita J 2008 The application of tooth temperature measurement in endodontic diagnosis: a review *J. Endod.* **34** 1435–40
[46] Bender B 2000 Reversible and irreversible painful pulpitides: diagnosis and treatment *Aust. Endod. J.* **26** 10–4
[47] Mumford J M 1967 Thermal and electrical stimulation of teeth in the diagnosis of pulpal and periapical disease *Proc. R. Soc. Med.* **60** 197–200
[48] Penna K J and Sadoff R S 1995 Simplified approach to use of electrical pulp tester *N. Y. State Dent. J.* **61** 30–1
[49] Cailleteau J G and Ludington J R 1989 Using the electric pulp tester with gloves: a simplified approach *J. Endodontics* **15** 80–1
[50] Kleier D J, Sexton J R and Averbach R E 1982 Electronic and clinical comparison of pulp testers *J. Dent. Res.* **61** 1413–5
[51] Ehrmann E H 1977 Pulp testers and pulp testing with particular reference to the use of dry ice *Aust. Dent. J.* **22** 272–9
[52] Närhi M, Virtanen A, Kuhta J and Huopaniemi T 1979 Electrical stimulation of teeth with a pulp tester in the cat *Scand. J. Dent. Res.* **87** 32–8
[53] Matthews B, Horiuchi H and Greenwood F 1974 The effects of stimulus polarity and electrode area on the threshold to monopolar stimulation of teeth in human subjects, with some preliminary observations on the use of a bipolar pulp tester *Arch. Oral Biol.* **19** 35–42
[54] Sui H, Lv Y, Xiao M, Zhou L, Qiao F, Zheng J, Sun C, Fu J, Chen Y and Liu Y 2021 Relationship between the difference in electric pulp test values and the diagnostic type of pulpitis *BMC Oral Health* **21** 339
[55] Dean J A and Sanders B J 2021 Treatment of deep caries, vital pulp exposure, and Nonvital teeth *McDonald and Avery's Dentistry for the Child and Adolescent* ed J A Dean, J E Jones, L A W Vinson, B J Sanders and J F Yepes (Amsterdam: Elsevier) pp 266–85
[56] Bender I B 2000 Pulpal pain diagnosis—a review *J. Endod.* **26** 175–9
[57] Woolley L H, Woodworth J and Dobbs J L 1974 A preliminary evaluation of the effects of electrical pulp testers on dogs with artificial pacemakers *J. Am. Dent. Assoc.* **89** 1099–101
[58] Luker J 1982 The pacemaker patient in the dental surgery *J. Dent.* **10** 326–32

[59] Miller C S, Leonelli F M and Latham E 1998 Selective interference with pacemaker activity by electrical dental devices *Oral Surg. Oral Med. Oral Pathol. Oral Radiol. Endod.* **85** 33–6

[60] Wilson B L, Broberg C, Baumgartner J C, Harris C and Kron J 2006 Safety of electronic apex locators and pulp testers in patients with implanted cardiac pacemakers or cardioverter/defibrillators *J. Endodontics* **32** 847–52

[61] Lizmar D, Veitía E, Acevedo A M and Rojas F 2010 Métodos convencionales y no convencionales para la detección de lesión inicial de caries *Rev. Bibliogr. Acta Odontol. Venez.* **49** 43–4

[62] Cueto R V 2009 Diagnóstico y tratamiento de lesiones cariosas incipientes en caras oclusales *Odontoestomatología* **11** 4–15

[63] Mohanraj M, Prabhu V R and Senthil R 2016 Diagnostic methods for early detection of dental caries—a review *Int. J. Pedod. Rehabil.* **1** 29–36

[64] Astvaldsdóttir A, Ahlund K, Holbrook W P, de Verdier B and Tranæus S 2012 Approximal caries detection by DIFOTI: *in vitro* comparison of diagnostic accuracy/Efficacy with film and digital radiography *Int. J. Dent.* **2012** 326401

[65] Laitala M L, Piipari L, Sämpi N, Korhonen M, Pesonen P, Joensuu T and Anttonen V 2017 Validity of digital imaging of fiber-optic transillumination in caries detection on proximal tooth surfaces *Int. J. Dent.* **2017** 8289636

[66] Macey R, Walsh T, Riley P, Hogan R, Glenny A M, Worthington H V, Clarkson J E and Ricketts D 2021 Transillumination and optical coherence tomography for the detection and diagnosis of enamel caries *Cochrane Database Syst. Rev.* **1** CD013855

[67] Bin-Shuwaish M, Yaman P, Dennison J and Neiva G 2008 The Correlation of DIFOTI to Clinical and Radiographic Images in Class II Carious Lesions *J. Am. Dent. Assoc.* **139** 1374–81

[68] Baltacioglu I H and Orhan K 2017 Comparison of diagnostic methods for early interproximal caries detection with near-infrared light transillumination: an *in vivo* study *BMC Oral Health* **17** 130

[69] Abdelaziz M and Krejci I 2014 DIAGNOcam—a near infrared digital imaging transillumination (NIDIT) technology *Int. J. Esthet. Dent.* **10** 158–65

[70] Ekstrand K R, Ricketts D N and Kidd E A 1997 Reproducibility and accuracy of three methods for assessment of demineralization depth of the occlusal surface: an *in vitro* examination *Caries Res.* **31** 224–31

[71] Kühnisch J, Söchtig F, Pitchika V, Laubender R, Neuhaus K W, Lussi A and Hickel R 2015 *in vivo* validation of near-infrared light transillumination for interproximal dentin caries detection *Clin. Oral Investig.* **20** 821–9

[72] Ozkan G and Guzel K 2017 Clinical evaluation of near-infrared light transillumination in approximal dentin caries detection *Lasers Med. Sci.* **32** 1417–22

[73] Bussaneli D, Restrepo M, Boldieri T, Pretel H, Mancini M, Santos-Pinto L and Cordeiro R 2015 Assessment of a new infrared laser transillumination technology (808 nm) for the detection of occlusal caries—an *in vitro* study *Lasers Med. Sci.* **30** 1873–9

[74] Abogazalah N, Eckert J G and Ando M 2017 *In vitro* performance of near infrared light transillumination at 780-nm and digital radiography for detection of non cavitated approximal caries *J. Dent.* **63** 44–50

[75] Söchtig F, Hickel R and Kühnisch J 2014 Caries detection and diagnostics with near-infrared light transillumination: clinical experiences *Quintessence Int.* **45** 531–8

[76] Elhennawy K, Askar H, Jost-Brinkmann P-G, Reda S, Al-Abdi A, Paris S and Schwendicke F 2018 In vitro performance of the DIAGNOcam for detecting proximal carious lesions adjacent to composite restorations *J. Dent.* **72** 39–43

[77] Melo M, Pascual A, Camps I, Ata-Ali F and Ata-Ali J 2019 Combined Near-Infrarred Light Transillumination and Direct Digital Radiography Increases Diagnostic In Approximal Caries *Sci. Rep.* **9** 14224

[78] Hsieh Y S, Ho Y C, Lee S Y, Chuang C C, Tsai J C, Lin K F and Sun C W 2013 Dental optical coherence tomography *Sensors* **13** 8928–49

[79] Huang D, Swanson E A, Lin C P, Schuman J S, Stinson W G, Chang W, Hee M R, Flotte T, Gregory K and Puliafito C A 1991 Optical coherence tomography *Science* **254** 1178–81

[80] Maciej W 2010 High-speed optical coherence tomography: basics and applications *Appl. Opt.* **49** D30–61

[81] Machoy M, Seeliger J, Szyszka-Sommerfeld L, Koprowski R, Gedrange T and Woźniak K 2017 The use of optical coherence tomography in dental diagnostics: a state-of-the-art review *J. Healthc. Eng.* **2017** 7560645

[82] Katkar R A, Tadinada S A, Amaechi B T and Fried D 2018 Optical coherence tomography *Dent. Clin. N. Am.* **62** 421–34

[83] Shimada Y, Yoshiyama M, Tagami J and Sumi Y 2020 Evaluation of dental caries, tooth crack, and age-related changes in tooth structure using optical coherence tomography *Jpn. Dent. Sci. Rev.* **56** 109–18

[84] Nakagawa H, Sadr A, Shimada Y, Tagami J and Sumi Y 2013 Validation of swept source optical coherence tomography (SS-OCT) for the diagnosis of smooth surface caries *in vitro J. Dent.* **41** 80–9

[85] Shimada Y, Sadr A, Burrow M F, Tagami J, Ozawa N and Sumi Y 2010 Validation of swept-source optical coherence tomography (SS-OCT) for the diagnosis of occlusal caries *J. Dent.* **38** 655–65

[86] Rochlen G K and Wolff M S 2011 Technological advances in caries diagnosis *Dent. Clin. N. Am.* **55** 441

[87] Ricketts D N, Kidd E A, Liepins P J and Wilson R F 1996 Histological validation of electrical resistance measurements in the diagnosis of occlusal caries *Caries Research* **30** 148–55

[88] Tassery H *et al* 2013 Use of new minimum intervention dentistry technologies in caries management *Aust. Dent. J.* **58** 40–59

[89] Longbottom C and Huysmans M C 2004 Electrical measurements for use in caries clinical trials *J. Dent. Res.* **83** C76–79

[90] Neuhaus K W, Longbottom C, Ellwood R and Lussi A 2009 Novel lesion detection aids *Monogr. Oral Sci.* **21** 52–62

[91] Gomez J, Tellez M, Pretty I A, Ellwood R P and Ismail A 2012 Non-cavitated carious lesions detection methods: a systematic review *Community Dent. Oral Epidemiol.* **41** 55–66

[92] Cortes D F, Ellwood R P and Ekstrand K R 2003 An *in vitro* comparison of a combined FOTI/visual examination of occlusal caries with other caries diagnostic methods and the effect of stain on their diagnostic performance *Caries Res.* **37** 8–16

[93] Huysmans M C and Longbottom C 2004 The challenges of validating diagnostic methods and selecting appropriate gold standards *J. Dent. Res.* **83** C48–52

[94] Fontana M and González-Cabezas C 2013 Exploring your technology options for detection of caries lesions *Inside Dent.* **9** https://www.aegisdentalnetwork.com/id/2013/03/technology-options-detection-caries-lesions

[95] Guimerà A, Calderón E, Los P and Christie A M 2008 Method and device for bio-impedance measurement with hard-tissue applications *Physiol. Meas.* **29** S279–90

[96] Pitts N, Longbottom C, Hall A F, Agnieszka C-W, Przemysław Ł, Masalski M, Przemyslaw B and Alasdair C 2008 Diagnostic accuracy of an Optimised AC impedance device to aid caries detection and monitoring *Caries Res.* **42** 185

[97] Renata C, Dominika P, Ilona W-C, Joanna Z and Teresa B 2013 AC-impedance spectroscopy and caries detection *Curr. Issues Pharm. Med. Sci.* **26** 344–6

[98] Macey R, Walsh T, Riley P, Glenny A M, Worthington H V, Clarkson J E and Ricketts D 2021 Electrical conductance for the detection of dental caries *Cochrane Database Syst. Rev.* **3** CD014547

[99] Lussi A and Francescut P 2003 Performance of conventional and new methods for the detection of occlusal caries in deciduous teeth *Caries Res.* **37** 2–7

[100] Lussi A, Zimmerli B, Hellwig E and Jaeggi T 2006 Influence of the condition of the adjacent tooth surface on fluorescence measurements for the detection of approximal caries *Eur. J. Oral Sci.* **114** 478–82

[101] Francescut P and Lussi A 2003 Correlation between fissure discoloration, diagnodent measurements, and caries depth: an *in vitro* study *Pediatr. Dent.* **25** 559–64

[102] Lussi A, Megert B, Longbottom C, Reich E and Francescut P 2001 Clinical performance of a laser fluorescence device for detection of occlusal caries lesions *Eur. J. Oral Sci.* **109** 14–9

[103] lussi A, Hibst R and Paulus R 2004 Diagnodent: an optical method for caries detection *J. Dent. Res.* **83** 80–3

[104] Bader J and Shugars D A 2004 A systematic review of the performance of a laser fluorescence device for detecting caries *J. Am. Dent. Assoc.* **135** 1413–26

[105] Strassler H E and Sensi L G 2008 Technology-enhanced caries detection and diagnosis *Compend. Contin. Educ. Dent.* **29** 464–5 468, 470

[106] Rodrigues J A, Hug I, Neuhaus K W and Lussi A 2011 Light-emitting diode and laser fluorescence-based devices in detecting occlusal caries *J. Biomed. Opt.* **16** 107003-1–105

[107] Diniz M B, Rodrigues J A and Lussi A 2012 Traditional and novel caries detection methods *Contemporary Approach to Dental Caries* ed M-Y Li (London: IntechOpen Limited) 6 105–28

[108] Guerrieri A, Gaucher C, Bonte E and Lasfargues J J 2012 Minimal intervention dentistry: part 4 detection and diagnosis of initial caries lesions *Br. Dent. J.* **213** 551–7

[109] Jablonski-Momeni A, Stucke J, Steinberg T and Heinzel-Gutenbrunner M 2012 Use of ICDAS-II, fluorescence-based methods, and radiography in detection and treatment decision of occlusal caries lesions: an *in vitro* study *Int. J. Dent.* **2012** 371595

[110] Tomczyk J, Komarnitki J, Zalewska M, Lekszycki T and Olczak-Kowalczyk D 2014 Fluorescence methods (VistaCam iX proof and DIAGNODent pen) for the detection of occlusal carious lesions in teeth recovered from archaeological context *Am. J. Phys. Anthropol.* **154** 525–34

[111] Terrer E, Koubi S, Dionne A, Weisrock G, Sarraquigne C, Mazuir A and Tassery H 2009 A new concept in restorative dentistry: light-induced fluorescence evaluator for diagnosis and treatment. Part 1: diagnosis and treatment of initial occlusal caries *J. Contemp. Dent. Prac.* **10** E086–E94

[112] Terrer E, Raskin A, Koubi S, Dionne A, Weisrock G, Sarraquigne C, Mazuir A and Tassery H 2010 A new concept in restorative dentistry: LIFEDT-light-induced fluorescence evaluator for diagnosis and treatment. Part 2: treatment of dentinal caries *J. Contemp. Dent. Prac.* **11** E095–102

[113] Zeitouny M, Feghali M, Nasr A, Abou-Samra P, Saleh N, Bourgeois D and Farge P 2014 SOPROLIFE System: An Accurate Diagnostic Enhancer *Sci. World J.* **2014** 1–8

[114] Lennon A M, Buchalla W, Rassner B, Becker K and Attin T 2006 Efficiency of 4 caries excavation methods compared *Oper. Dent.* **31** 551–5

[115] Lennon A M, Attin T, Martens S and Buchalla W 2009 Fluorescence aided caries excavation, caries detector, and conventional caries excavation in primary teeth *Pediatr. Dent.* **31** 316–9

[116] Ten B J 1996 Light scattering and related methods in caries diagnosis; G Stookey *Proc. 1st Annual Indiana Conf.: Early Detection of Dental Caries* (Indianapolis, IN: Indiana University School of Dentistry) pp 81–90

[117] Stookey G K 2005 Quantitative light fluorescence: a technology for early monitoring of the caries process *Dent. Clin. N. Am.* **49** 753–70

[118] Amaechi B T and Higham S M 2002 Quantitative light-induced fluorescence: A potential tool for general dental assessment *J. Biomed. Opt.* **7** 7–13

[119] Alammari M R, Smith P W, de Josselin de Jong E and Higham S M 2013 Quantitative light-induced fluorescence (QLF): A tool for early occlusal dental caries detection and supporting decision making in vivo *J. Dent.* **41** 127–32

[120] Mandelis A, Nicolaides L, Feng C and Abrams S H 2000 Novel dental depth profilometric imaging using simultaneous frequency-domain infrared photothermal radiometry and laser luminescence *Proc. SPIE* **3916** 130–7

[121] Nicolaides L, Mandelis A and Abrams S H 2000 Novel dental dynamic depth profilometric imaging using simultaneous frequency-domain infrared photothermal radiometry and laser luminescence *J. Biomed. Opt.* **5** 31–9

[122] Jeon R J, Han C, Mandelis A, Sanchez V and Abrams S H 2004 Diagnosis of pit and fissure caries using frequencydomain infrared photothermal radiometry and modulated laser luminescence *Caries Res.* **38** 497–513

[123] Jeon R J, Matvienko A, Mandelis A, Abrams S H, Amaechi B T and Kulkarni G 2007 Detection of interproximal demineralized lesions on human teeth *in vitro* using frequency-domain infrared photothermal radiometry and modulated luminescence *J. Biomed. Opt.* **034028**

[124] Garcia J A, Mandelis A, Abrams S H and Matvienko A 2013 Photothermal radiometry and modulated luminescence: applications for dental caries detection *Handbook of Biophotonics* (Hoboken, NJ: Wiley) 1047–52

[125] Silvertown J D *et al* 2017 Multi-centre clinical evaluation of photothermal radiometry and luminescence correlated with international benchmarks for caries detection *Open Dent. J.* **11** 636–47

[126] Jeon R J, Mandelis A, Sanchez V and Abrams S H 2004 Nonintrusive, noncontacting frequency-domain photothermal radiometry and luminescence depth profilometry of carious and artificial subsurface lesions in human *J. Biomed. Opt.* **9** 804–19

[127] Mandelis A, Abrams S, Jeon J S, Kulkarni K and Matvienko A 2012 *Method and apparatus using infrared photothermal radiometry (PTR) and modulated laser luminescence (LUM)*

for diagnostics of defects in teeth US 8,306,608 inventors: Quantum Dental Technologies Inc https://image-ppubs.uspto.gov/dirsearch-public/print/downloadPdf/8306608
[128] The Canary System https://thecanarysystem.com/about.php. (accessed 19 January 2023)
[129] Macey R, Walsh T, Riley P, Glenny A M, Worthington H V, Fee P A, Clarkson J E and Ricketts D 2020 Fluorescence devices for the detection of dental caries *Cochrane Database Syst. Rev.* **12** CD013811
[130] Gimenez T, Braga M M, Raggio D P, Deery C, Ricketts D N and Mendes F M 2013 Fluorescence-based methods for detecting caries lesions: systematic review, meta-analysis and sources of heterogeneity *PLoS One* **8** e60421
[131] Nekoofar M H, Ghandi M M, Hayes S J and Dummer P M 2006 The fundamental operating principles of electronic root canal length measurement devices *Int. Endodont. J.* **39** 595–609
[132] Ebrahim A K, Wadachi R and Suda H 2007 Electronic apex locators—a review *J. Med. Dent. Sci.* **54** 125–36
[133] Gordon M P and Chandler N P 2004 Electronic apex locators *Int. Endod. J.* **37** 425–37
[134] Juerchott A, Pfefferle T, Flechtenmacher C, Mente J, Bendszus M, Heiland S and Hilgenfeld T 2018 Differentiation of periapical granulomas and cysts by using dental MRI: a pilot study *Int. J. Oral Sci.* **10** 17
[135] Heggie J C P 2001 Magnetic resonance imaging: principles, methods and techniques by perry sprawls *Australas. Phys. Eng. Sci. Med.* **24** 57
[136] Ariji Y, Ariji E, Nakashima M and Iohara K 2018 Magnetic resonance imaging in endodontics: a literature review *Oral Radiol.* **34** 10–6
[137] Starkoff B 2014 Ultrasound physical principles in today's technology *Australas. J. Ultrasound Med.* **17** 4–10
[138] Aggarwal V and Singla M 2010 Use of computed tomography scans and ultrasound in differential diagnosis and evaluation of nonsurgical management of periapical lesions *Oral Surg. Oral Med. Oral Pathol. Oral Radiol. Endod.* **109** 917–23
[139] Natanasabapathy V, Arul B, Mishra A, Varghese A, Padmanaban S, Elango S and Arockiam S 2021 Ultrasound imaging for the differential diagnosis of periapical lesions of endodontic origin in comparison with histopathology—a systematic review and meta-analysis *Int. Endodont. J.* **54** 693–711
[140] Raghav N, Reddy S S, Giridhar A G, Murthy S, Yashodha Devi B K, Santana N, Rakesh N and Kaushik A 2010 Comparison of the efficacy of conventional radiography, digital radiography, and ultrasound in diagnosing periapical lesions *Oral Surg. Oral Med. Oral Pathol. Oral Radiol. Endod.* **110** 379–85

Chapter 3

Complementary physical methods for the detection of carious lesions

Douglas Roberto Monteiro, Caio Sampaio, Beatriz Diaz Fabregat, Wilmer Ramirez Carmona, Evelyn Carmo Oliveira, Guilherme dos Santos Gomes Alves and Juliano Pelim Pessan

Dental caries is a biofilm-dependent disease, resulting from the slow but progressive mineral loss from tooth structures caused by exposure to fermentable carbohydrates. The occlusal and approximal surfaces are often the most affected tooth sites for caries development due to their intrinsic stagnation sites, which facilitate biofilm accumulation and hinder the action of salivary buffers. The intricate anatomy of the occlusal surfaces, which includes pits and fissures, makes the detection of early lesions by visual and tactile inspection a difficult process, often involving unnecessary dental destruction due to false positive detection. Likewise, the detection of approximal lesions may sometimes be unfeasible by conventional clinical examination. Considering that accurate early detection is paramount for the prevention of further tooth destruction, increasing interest has been targeted at diagnostic tools that can be used alone or in association with conventional visual–tactile approaches. This chapter presents and discusses diagnostic tools based on physical principles, including conventional and digital intraoral radiography, laser fluorescence, quantitative light-induced fluorescence, fiber-optic transillumination (FOTI), and cone beam computed tomography. The physical principles of each method, their main advantages and disadvantages, and the available scientific evidence are addressed for each method.

3.1 Introduction

Dental caries is one of the main oral diseases, affecting individuals of all ages worldwide, and is characterized by demineralization of the mineral content of dental tissues (enamel and dentin) and by the degradation of dentin proteins. It is a sucrose-dependent disease, mediated by the dental biofilm, presenting a multifactorial etiology. Imbalance in the etiological factors, along with oral environmental and personal

doi:10.1088/978-0-7503-5316-8ch3

factors, may lead to the rapid destruction of dental hard tissues. On the other hand, the high availability of fluoride products for community and professional use, along with self-application vehicles, has led to significant changes in the pattern of disease development, particularly those related to the longer progression time of the lesions and the hypermineralization of the surface layer of the initial enamel lesions (Struzycka 2014, Simón-Soro *et al* 2015, Pitts *et al* 2017, Machiulskiene *et al* 2020, Tinanoff *et al* 2019).

The diagnosis of caries disease is a complex process, since caries can present themselves as very small, non-cavitated enamel lesions or even as subclinical enamel lesions, which can further progress to extensive lesions in the dentin. Traditional methods, such as visual and tactile examination, sometimes associated with radiographic examination, are most commonly used by dental professionals. In this sense, it is worth noting that the radiographic examination is performed by detecting carious lesions through imaging resources of the regions of interest, while the diagnosis of the disease involves joint interpretation of the data obtained during the patient's anamnesis and the proper interpretation of clinical and radiographic data. Thus, the diagnosis of the disease—and not only lesion detection—is essential to guide the clinical conduct of the professional. For this reason, the radiographic examination is considered complementary to the tactile–visual examination, with the aim of identifying the presence or absence of disease or aggravation, providing information about the nature and extent of the disease, and enabling the formation of differential diagnoses (Nyvad 2004, Pretty 2006).

Tactile–visual detection methods aim to identify the presence of initial lesions, since they allow for the observation of aspects of normality or alterations related to texture, brightness, and color. However, these methods have limitations in terms of sensitivity and specificity as well as low precision on occlusal and proximal surfaces. Such limitations have driven the development of new technologies that allow the measurement of small changes in dental tissues compared to healthy tissue (Nyvad 2004, Murdoch-Kinch and McLean 2003). Such methods must meet certain criteria in order to be considered adequate, including reliability, non-invasiveness, the ability to detect carious lesions in their early stages with differentiation between reversible and irreversible lesions, affordable cost, comfort for the patient, easy execution, and effectiveness for all surfaces of the teeth (Pretty 2006).

This chapter aims to present the main auxiliary methods that can be used as a complement to visual inspection, which include conventional and digital intraoral radiographic examinations, laser fluorescence, quantitative light-induced fluorescence, FOTI, and cone beam computed tomography. The physical principles of each method, its main advantages and disadvantages, and the available scientific evidence are addressed for each method.

3.2 Radiographic examinations

3.2.1 History and background

The radiographic examination, popularly known as an x-ray, is characterized by electromagnetic radiation which involves the confluence of a magnetic field with an electric field; this radiation propagates in vacuum, transporting energy (Dyson 1990). This diagnostic tool is the method most used in daily dental practice, along with the tactile–visual clinical examination.

In brief, x-rays were discovered by the German physicist Wilhelm Conrad Röntgen, and their name ('X') represented the unknown variable, as the phenomenon was hitherto unknown. In November 1895, during a study of cathode ray luminescence in a Crookes tube, he noticed a glow projected on a phosphor plate; even after an aluminum foil was placed between the plate and the tube, the glow remained. With this evidence, he carried out his first experiment with the help of his wife, Anna Bertha Roentgen, who placed her hand on a photographic film and, after a few minutes of exposure to the unknown rays from the device, an image of the bones and soft parts of her hand was produced (Kotzur 1994, Dyson 1990).

After this experiment, Röntgen verified that materials with low density, such as muscles, are traversed by x-rays, while materials with high density, such as bone, absorb the rays (due to the Compton effect), thus confirming the theory of his observations. This was considered to be the first radiography known to history (Kotzur 1994, Dyson 1990). Between the years 1922–45, his carefully detailed study was consolidated following advances in studies related to the interpretation of the energy of atoms; subsequently, x-ray tubes began to be developed (Kotzur 1994). The development of the applications and potential consequences of the use of x-rays has intensified from 1945 to the present day. Today, more than 100 years after its discovery, the ionizing radiation used in x-ray equipment has given rise to new technologies, such as computed tomography, digital x-rays, magnetic resonance imaging, and mammography (Webb 1990, Christie and Tansey 2006).

3.2.2 Radiation physics

The principle of x-ray generation is based on the use of a given voltage at high speed, so that thermoelectrons produced at the cathode collide with the anode to obtain continuous rays, which are capable of generating ionization and excitation (Young 1999, Hewitt 2001). Ionizing radiation, therefore, is the energy transmitted through waves in a space or medium, and its energy is superior to the binding of electrons to the nucleus. It is classified as: 'primary radiation' when direct ionizing radiation is charged with sufficient kinetic energy to ionize atoms and molecules by collision, 'indirect radiation' when it is not charged with a high level of kinetic energy, 'secondary radiation' when electromagnetic radiation is propagated in the form of waves through the oscillation of electric and magnetic fields, and 'particle radiation,' which has high-velocity mass (Young 1999, Hewitt 2001).

Photons and neutrons release a discrete number of ions during their interaction with matter, so that the process of matter ionization begins when the released electrons and ions are stopped. The passage of ionizing radiation produces ionization, excitation, and radiation; these exchanges lead to changes in physical and chemical properties, which also result in a change in the amount of radiation produced, whether in inert or biological materials (Feynman *et al* 2006, Hubbell 2006, Turner 2004, Evans 1955, Young 1999, Hewitt 2001).

X-radiation is invisible and cannot be detected by any of the human senses. It also has no weight or mass; it propagates at the speed of light and in a straight line and is capable of being deflected and scattered. Furthermore, it always diverges from a point, being able to penetrate or pass through the materials according to their composition, which may generate biological changes in living cells (Young 1999, Hewitt 2001).

3.2.3 Radiographic films

Radiographic films are composed of a polyester base covered by a double layer of emulsion, which coats the polyester base on both sides; silver halogen salts (bromides or silver halides) are used in the emulsion and are responsible for the image production of radiographic films. A very thin gelatin-based protective layer covers this entire set, protecting the film against excessive handling (Brown *et al* 1973).

Radiographic films are still the main device for recording images; therefore, recognizing their constitution is useful for their correct use and in order to obtain a quality image. The polyester base has very specific characteristics, being produced of a plastic material which cannot be dissolved in a liquid medium. It needs to be rigid and thin, so that it fits in the patient's mouth. It should also be translucent so that it is visible on a negatoscope, and, as a safety measure, it should be fire retardant (Hardman *et al* 1987, Hedin 1989). The emulsion has two layers and is formed of a silver salt, either silver halide or bromide, and does not dissolve in a liquid medium. The x-rays sensitize the silver granules so that after the film is exposed, bromine or a halide is formed, thus creating a latent image (Hardman *et al* 1987, Hedin 1989, Ludlow 1997).

As previously mentioned, the protective layer is intended to protect the emulsion from excessive handling at the time of radiography, preventing the radiograph from becoming smudged. The film is encased in a protective black paper wrapper (to protect against light) and then in an outer white paper or plastic wrapping (to protect it from contamination by the patient's fluids) and a lead sheet, the latter being responsible for providing rigidity to the film assembly and protecting against secondary radiation, which occurs, for example, when the light beam strikes a soft tissue, displacing electron beams and producing a secondary image. The lead sheet also helps to identify a film exposure error in cases in which it is exposed to x-rays by mistake. In this case, it is noteworthy that lead invalidates the image because, due to its high molecular weight, it will absorb the rays, and the resulting x-ray will lack contrast and sharpness. After sensitization, the film undergoes chemical processing to produce a two-dimensional image of the structures of interest. A dark chamber (portable or automatic) is needed for the chemical processing, which involves chemicals such as as a developer and a fixer.

According to White and Pharoah (2004), films can be classified according to their use, size, number of pellicles, and sensitivity. In terms of size, extraoral films vary according to the purpose of the radiograph (typically measuring 13×18, 18×24, 12×30, or 15×30 cm). On the other hand, intraoral films are measured in inches, with sizes ranging from zero to four: the size zero is for small children (22×35 mm); size one is relatively narrow and is used for views of the anterior teeth (24×40 mm); size two is the standard film size used for adults (31×41 mm); and type three (57×76 mm) is used for occlusal takes. In terms of the number of films in each envelope, they are classified as single or double, respectively, when the envelope contains one or two films. As for sensitivity (D, E, F), the higher the letter, the more sensitive the film is to x-rays, and the more sensitive the film, the smaller the amount of radiation needed to produce an image. The sensitivity largely depends on the size and shape of the silver granules, that is, the larger the silver granules, the more sensitive they are to x-rays.

Contrast and density are also important characteristics to be considered; the specific contrast of the radiographic colors (black, white, and gray) is influenced by the voltage of the equipment; the higher the voltage, the greater the contrast (and the quality) of the radiograph. At high contrast, the image is either too white or too black, while gray colors prevail for low contrast. Therefore, ideal radiographs are obtained at medium contrast; white, black, and the intermediate shades of gray then generate an outline of restorations and anatomical structures, so that the contours are also a property of the radiographic film and are directly related to its granulation. The smaller the silver grains, the greater the detail or definition of an image. Density, on the other hand, is characterized by the darkening of the image, so the longer the exposure time, the darker the radiograph. Contrast and density are related, because if the contrast is inadequate, the density will also be compromised (Hardman *et al* 1987, Hedin 1989, Ludlow 1997).

3.2.4 Intraoral conventional radiography

The simultaneous production of a clear picture of both dental and adjacent structures is considered to be the main advantage of conventional radiography. This type of examination involves administering a low dose of radiation to the patient and requires relatively low-cost equipment and supplies (Basting and Serra 1999, Nyvad *et al* 1999, Braga *et al* 2010, Nyvad 2004). The poor coverage of the oral surfaces, on the other hand, is one of its disadvantages, as a complete examination of all teeth requires several x-rays to be taken. In addition, this technique is not recommended for patients with trismus and those who have strong nausea reflexes. Despite such drawbacks, conventional radiography is still the most widely used image-based examination in the dental routine. Bitewing and periapical exams are the most widely used modalities of intraoral conventional radiography for caries detection and assessments of lesion depth, as described in more details below.

3.2.4.1 The interproximal technique (bitewing)

The interproximal technique, or bitewing, is used as an auxiliary method for caries detection (especially for approximal lesions), the determination of lesion depth and its relationship with dental pulp, the evaluation of crown and bone integrity, and the assessment of approximal restorations and prosthetic crowns. This technique is considered to be highly sensitive, which is the reason that it is widely used in the dental routine. In this technique, dental enamel mineral loss can be detected by radiolucency, similarly to excesses of restorative materials in dental restorations (Hintze *et al* 1998). When radiolucency is verified in the inner portion of the dentin, a visual inspection may well have detected the lesion; conversely, when radiolucency is verified in the outer portion of the dentin, the probability of cavitation ranges from 41% to 79% (Hintze *et al* 1998, Wenzel 2004).

3.2.4.2 Periapical radiography

The periapical technique is essentially used for analyzing one tooth or a group of teeth from the apex to the crown, as well as the supporting structures, especially those related to the dental periapical status (Nair *et al* 1999, Musri *et al* 2021). The natural inclination of the teeth in their axis (in the alveolar bone) must be considered before a radiographic exposure is made in order to meet the ideal requirements of the technique. This implies that the professional must be knowledgeable in dental anatomy and root angulation, especially when the technique is not performed using a positioner (Antony *et al* 2020).

The indications for periapical radiography include large coronal carious lesions, inflammation or periapical infection, dental trauma, and evaluation of the root morphology and position prior to extraction (Foster Page *et al* 2018, Bourguignon *et al* 2020). Despite the versatility of the technique, some limitations should be mentioned. This technique is not capable of delimiting large lesions and detecting proximal or incipient carious lesions; the bitewing technique is the most appropriate for such purposes (Foster Page *et al* 2018).

In brief, the periapical technique can be used in two ways: the parallelism technique, which requires that the long axes of the tooth and of the radiographic film are positioned parallel to each other, so that the main x-ray beam is perpendicularly incident (90° angle) to both; and the bisector technique, which is used when parallelism between the long axis of the tooth and of the radiographic film is not possible; in this scenario, the main x-ray beam is perpendicularly incident (90° angle) to the bisector plane between the long axis of the tooth and the radiographic film (Antony *et al* 2020).

3.2.5 Digital radiography

With the advent of more advanced technologies, digital radiography has emerged from its conventional (analog) version. In this modality, the radiographic pellicle is replaced by sensors that transfer the captured information directly to a computer, where the images are transformed into digital images and then displayed on a monitor (Ricketts *et al* 2007). This is very useful for clinicians, as they can determine that either no change in the tooth structure has occurred (when the result of subtraction is zero), or changes in its constitution have occurred (a value different from zero after subtraction). Digital radiography is, therefore, a valuable tool for the diagnosis of primary and secondary caries, especially in follow-up consultations, in which the procedure requires the effective registration of the lesion (Ricketts *et al* 2007).

One of the main advantages of this technique is the easy manipulation of the images, which allows the subtraction of shades of gray between two images. The procedure is also much less time-consuming than its analog counterpart, as the image is available immediately after the radiographic exposure. Furthermore, it is more eco-friendly and less hazardous to the professionals, as it does not involve the use of chemicals for image processing. Despite these and other advantages of digital radiography, a systematic review of this issue concluded that not all of the claimed advantages of digital radiography were actually confirmed in clinical practice. Patient discomfort as well as error and repetition rates were found to be higher for digital radiography (Wenzel and Møystad 2010).

As for the reduction in radiation dose—one of the most claimed advantages of digital radiography—the same review showed that no difference could be evidenced regarding the reduction in radiation dose (Wenzel and Møystad 2010). Since then, advances on this topic have emerged due to the advent of new technologies and the rapid evolution of the existing facilities. Today, strategies for increasing image sharpness and quality are even more advanced in terms of detection and interpretation (Wenzel 2021). Thus, with the shift from analog to digital radiography, the dose of radiation required for each exposure has substantially decreased (Chauhan and Wilkins 2019).

Evidence to attest the differences in the detection capacity of these two methods is scarce. Overall, comparisons between the two techniques have been most often explored for interproximal carious lesions. For approximal caries, sensitivity values of 0.32 (0.26–0.38) were reported for the conventional technique (ultraspeed film), and of 0.35 (0.28–0.41), 0.38 (0.32–0.44), and 0.34 (0.28–0.40) for three other digital methods (Dexis, Dexis+, and Digora, respectively). In addition, specificity values of 0.94 (0.92–0.96), 0.96 (0.95–0.98), 0.97 (0.95–0.98), and 0.96 (0.94–0.97), respectively, were observed for conventional radiography, Dexis, Dexis+, and Digora. Positive and negative predilection values consisted respectively of 0.64 and 0.81 for ultraspeed film, 0.76 and 0.82 for Dexis, 0.79 and 0.82 for Dexis+, and 0.73 and 0.82 for Digora (Haak *et al* 2001). The authors concluded that conventional and digital radiography showed comparable results. Another study with similar aims reported sensitivities of 0.14 (0.047–0.328), 0.15 (0.031–0.297), 0.16 (0.047 0.281), and 0.16 (0.031 0.250), respectively for Digora blue plate, Digora white plate, DenOptix, and conventional radiography (Insight film) (Pontual *et al* 2010). Regarding specificity, values of 0.93 (0.830–1.000), 0.94 (0.874–1000), 0.89 (0.807–0.977), and 0.92 (0.818–1000), were reported for the four methods, respectively. As for accuracy, the corresponding values were 0.59 (0.559–0.632), 0.61 (0.556–0.649), 0.58 (0.546–0.632), and 0.60 (0.559–0.632), respectively. In line with the previous study, the authors concluded that the performances of the digital methods were similar to those of the analog versions and that the histological depth of enamel lesions was not correlated with the methods evaluated (Pontual *et al* 2010).

In addition, a recent study *in vitro* study of extracted human teeth compared the diagnostic accuracies of storage phosphor plates (digital radiography) and conventional films with a gold-standard stereomicroscope, observing the satisfactory diagnostic accuracy of conventional film and digital radiography in comparison to the stereomicroscope. The authors also found no statistical differences in the diagnostic accuracies of the two radiographic modalities (conventional film and digital radiography), given that neither outperformed the other in detecting interproximal caries (Vijayan *et al* 2022). Despite the lack of significant differences observed between the radiographic modalities, the authors suggested that digital radiography is preferable due to the lower dose required for the technique in comparison to that needed for analog radiography (Vijayan *et al* 2022).

In this sense, in light of the pros and cons of digital radiography in relation to conventional radiography, it is reasonable to consider that the choice of using the digital version depends on the clinician's personal opinion regarding costs and benefits (for both the patient and the professional), as the literature describes similar outcomes in terms of accuracy for both the conventional method and the digital method. Nonetheless, consideration should be given to the radiation dose administered by the modality chosen for use.

3.3 Fiber-optic transillumination

FOTI-based technology is one of the most recently studied tools for caries detection. In short, optical fiber consists of flexible cylindrical fibers based on glass or plastic of high optical quality. Due to the higher refractive index of the fiber core, the light rays are reflected back to the core, following a principle based on Snell's Law (the so-called total internal reflection) (Strassler and Pitel 2014). In recent years, this technology has been used for the detection of tumors, the evaluation of sinuses, and as an adjunct method for caries diagnosis (Sharan *et al* 2011).

Understanding the relationship between dental hard tissues and their optical properties can help us to comprehend how these technologies work. Sound enamel is based on densely packed hydroxyapatite crystals, i.e. a semitransparent structure, in contrast to the underlying dentin shade which is responsible for tooth coloration (Pretty 2006). For demineralized enamel (i.e. white-spot lesions), the penetrating photons are scattered, resulting in optical disruption, which makes the tooth visibly appear whiter. Although water has a similar refractive index to that of enamel, when this tissue is dried, the porous surface of demineralized enamel is filled by air, which has a lower refractive index than that of enamel; this is the reason that the lesions become more visible and clearer, even under visual examination. Optic transillumination technologies enhance these optical properties of enamel. In brief, light is directed through the tooth, and the scattering effect can be seen as shadows in the hard dental tissues.

FOTI devices for caries diagnosis have a series of strengths compared to other technologies, including low cost, safety, and simplicity of use (Côrtes *et al* 2003, Pretty 2006). Nonetheless, some drawbacks must also be considered. Firstly, FOTI comprises a subjective system, which means that the operator can be subject to bias, similarly to visual inspection. In addition, FOTI devices do not record the images obtained during examinations, which has important clinical implications for lesion monitoring (Schneiderman *et al* 1997, Pretty 2006). These limitations have stimulated the development of digital imaging fiber-optic transillumination (DIFOTI). The 'digital version' of FOTI allows the future assessment of images obtained during examination, which is very beneficial for planning purposes. However, even with such improvements, some limitations of FOTI have not been overcome by DIFOTI, as the examinations are still visual, meaning that the diagnostic process is based on the appearance of scattering, which still relies on the operator's precision and calibration (Pretty 2006).

Despite the aforementioned limitations, since the emergence of FOTI/DIFOTI, numerous studies have assessed the efficacy of these methods for caries diagnosis. Most of these studies have presented data on the specificity (SP) and sensibility (SE) of these methods (in addition to other important statistical parameters) for the detection of carious lesions on different dental surfaces. Sometimes, these studies considered the severity of the lesion or the type of dental tissue involved (e.g. cavitation, white-spot lesions, or caries at the enamel or dentin levels), presenting different outcomes for each parameter, which are further detailed below. Table 3.1 summarizes the available evidence on the effectiveness of FOTI and DIFOTI for caries detection.

Some studies, including systematic reviews, have addressed the accuracy of illumination technologies for the detection of carious lesions restricted to the enamel. Data from a recent *in vitro* study that aimed to compare visual examination with a visible-light transillumination method (using DIFOTI) using an occlusal view (DIFOTI-occl), an axial view (buccal and lingual: DIFOTI-axial), and a combination of all views (DIFOTI-all) for the diagnosis of non-cavitated carious lesions (NCCLs) showed sensitivities of 0.43, 0.86, 0.91, and 0.90 for DIFOTI-occlusal, DIFOTI-axial, DIFOTI-all, and for visual identification according to the International Caries Detection and Assessment System (ICDAS), respectively. The corresponding values for specificity were 0.75, 0.93, 0.69, and 0.83, respectively. The Spearman correlation coefficient between μ-CT and DIFOTI-occlusal was low ($r = 0.39$), while high correlation was observed between μ-CT and DIFOTI-axial ($r = 0.80$), DIFOTI-all ($r = 0.91$), and visual-ICDAS ($r = 0.90$). The authors suggested that DIFOTI performed better using the axial view in comparison to the occlusal view for the diagnosis of NCCLs (Abogazalah *et al* 2019). In spite of these associations of DiFOTI with the visual method in some views, it is important to highlight the *in vitro* nature of the study, which cannot be considered to be strong evidence.

In this sense, an interesting systematic review evaluated the performances of different tools for detecting NCCLs. The authors documented sensitivities of 0.17–0.96, 0.16–0.96, 0.12–0.84, 0.21–0.96, 0.61–0.92, and 0.82 for visual inspection, laser fluorescence or DIAGNOdent (DD), radiographic examination, FOTI, electrical conductance, and quantitative light-induced fluorescence, respectively. For specificity, values of 0.46–1.0, 0.25–1.00, 0.55–0.99, 0.74–0.88, 0.73–1.0, and 0.92 were obtained for visual inspection, laser fluorescence or DD, radiographic examination, FOTI, electrical conductance, and quantitative light-induced fluorescence, respectively. The authors concluded that visual methods remain the standard for caries detection in dental practice and that the diagnosis of NCCLs is more accurate when performed in combination with the visual method and the use of other strategies (Gomez *et al* 2013).

Following this rationale, a recent systematic review by the Cochrane collaboration estimated the diagnostic accuracy of different illumination tools for detecting

Table 3.1. Available evidence for the effectiveness of FOTI and DiFOTI for caries detection.

Author (year)	Aim	Protocol	Diagnostic tool(s)	Dental surface	Sensitivity/specificity/or statistical parameters	Main results/conclusions
Serban *et al* (2022)	To assess the diagnostic accuracy of emerging technologies in the diagnosis of dentin caries.	Systematic review	Laser fluorescence (LF), transillumination, light-emitting diode devices, optical coherence tomography (OCT), alternating current impedance spectroscopy, fluorescence cameras (FCs), photothermal radiometry, and modulated luminescence technology	Proximal and occlusal	Both for FOTI and near-infrared light transillumination (NIR-LT) there have been a very small number of studies.	Due to the limited number of studies included, further assessments are necessary to obtain strong results.
Walsh *et al* (2022)	To analyze the diagnostic accuracy of different technologies used to detect and inform the diagnosis of early caries using published Cochrane systematic reviews.	Analysis of systematic reviews	Fluorescence, visual or visual–tactile classification systems, imaging, transillumination, and electrical conductance or impedance	Not restricted (enamel)	Transillumination: sensitivity: 0.76 (0.63, 0.86) specificity: 0.82 (0.68, 0.91)	The greatest pairwise differences were observed in the summary sensitivity points for imaging and all other technologies, but the summary specificity points were broadly similar. Low certainty of evidence downgraded due to study limitations, inconsistency, and indirectness.

Macey *et al* (2021)	To estimate the diagnostic test accuracy of different illumination tests for the detection and diagnosis of enamel caries in children and adults.	Systematic review (Cochrane)	OCT, near-infrared (NIR), and fiber-optic technology	Not restricted (enamel)	There was a significant difference in the sensitivity of the different devices studied ($Chi^2(2) = 31.24$, $P < 0.01$) with a higher sensitivity of 0.94 (95% CI 0.88 to 0.97) for OCT compared to NIR 0.58 (95% CI 0.46 to 0.68) and FOTI/DIFOTI 0.47 (95% CI 0.35 to 0.59), but no meaningful difference in specificity ($Chi^2(2) = 3.47$, $P = 0.18$).	FOTI is a readily available and user-friendly tool; however, it shows limitations in its ability to detect enamel caries but may be considered successful in the identification of sound teeth.
Kapor *et al* (2021)	To assess the diagnostic performance of commonly used methods for occlusal caries diagnostics in relation to their ability to detect (dentin) caries *in vivo* and *in vitro*	Systematic review	Visual examination (VE), bitewing radiography (BW), LF, and FOTI	Occlusal	Data on DIFOTI: *In vivo*: insufficient data; *In vitro*: Caries detection level: sensitivity: 0.97 (−0.92 to 0.99); specificity: 0.50 (0.34–0.66); AUC: 0.92; DOR: 38.33 (10.15–144.77);	Insufficient data on the performance of DIFOTI in clinical conditions. VE, BW radiography, and LF provide acceptable measures for their diagnostic performance on occlusal surfaces.

(*Continued*)

Table 3.1. (*Continued*)

Author (year)	Aim	Protocol	Diagnostic tool(s)	Dental surface	Sensitivity/specificity/or statistical parameters	Main results/conclusions
					dentin detection level: sensitivity: 0.49 (0.20–0.79); specificity: 0.97 (0.89–0.994); AUC: 0.92; DOR: 37.77 (13.69–104.19).	
Antipoviene *et al* (2020)	To assess the depth of proximal carious lesions clinically detected using DIFOTI in comparison to periapical radiographs.	Clinical trial	Digital imaging transillumination (DIFOTI; DIAGNOcam™—KaVo) and periapical (PA) digital radiographs	Proximal	Not reported	DIFOTI and PA yielded different results regarding the scores of demineralization depth. PA had a tendency to record greater demineralization scores relative to DIFOTI: in 37% of cases, the recorded demineralization depth was higher according to PA, and in 26% of cases, the recorded demineralization depth was higher in the DIFOTI images.

Marmaneu-Menero *et al* (2020)	To analyze the available evidence for the validity of the transillumination method in the diagnosis of interproximal caries	Systematic review	DIFOTI and NIR-LT	Proximal	Sensitivity: 0.69 (confidence interval: 0.54–0.81); Specificity: 0.89 (confidence interval: 0.61–0.98); AUC: 0.79 with a confidence interval of 0.67–0.87.	There is no strong evidence to affirm that transillumination may fully replace x-rays in the complementary diagnosis of carious lesions. It is suggested that further studies should focus on the sensitivity and specificity of this method.
Tagliaferro *et al* (2019)	To assess practices related to the diagnosis of dental caries among dentists from a city in Brazil (Araraquara).	Observational study	Not applicable	Not restricted	Not applicable	Most of the subjects (dentists) reported they most commonly use visual, tactile, and radiographic imaging for the diagnosis of dental caries. Digital imaging transillumination is not very commonly used.
Abogazalah *et al* (2019)	To compare visual examination using ICDAS scores with a visible-light-transillumination method (using	*In vitro*	DIFOTI	Proximal	Sensitivity: DIFOTI-occlusal: 0.42, DIFOTI-axial: 0.86, DIFOTI-all: 0.91, and for ICDAS: 0.89.	It can be suggested that for the detection of non-cavitated approximal carious lesions, DIFOTI performs better using

(*Continued*)

Table 3.1. (*Continued*)

Author (year)	Aim	Protocol	Diagnostic tool(s)	Dental surface	Sensitivity/specificity/or statistical parameters	Main results/conclusions
	DIFOTI) using an occlusal view (DIFOTI-occl), an axial view (buccal and lingual: DIFOTI-axial), and a combination of all views (DIFOTI-all) in the detection of non-cavitated proximal caries.				Specificity: DIFOTI-occlusal: 0.75, DIFOTI-axial: 0.93, DIFOTI-all: 0.69, and for ICDAS: 0.83. Spearman correlation coefficients with μ-CT for DIFOTI-occlusal (r = 0.39) showed weak association, while DIFOTI-axial (r = 0.80), DIFOTI-all (r = 0.91), and ICDAS (r = 0.90) showed moderate association.	the axial view than the occlusal view.
Laitala *et al* (2017)	To evaluate the validity of the DIFOTI method in comparison with clinical visual (CV) examination and BW radiography in the detection of carious lesions on the proximal surfaces of teeth.	Clinical trial	VE, BW, and DIFOTI	Proximal	DIFOTI detected more initial and manifested carious lesions compared with CV examination and BW radiography. Of the analyzed tooth surfaces, 69.8% were classified as sound by DIFOTI, 80.3% by BW radiography, and	The DIFOTI method was demonstrated to be a potential tool for everyday clinical practice and presented promising trends in comparison to CV examination and BW radiography.

					91.6% by CV examination. Initial carious lesions were found in 21.2% of the surfaces by DIFOTI, in 14.1% by BW radiography, and in 6.2% by CV examination, whereas the proportions for manifested dental carious lesions were 9.0%, 5.6%, and 2.2%, respectively. The interexaminer agreement regarding the DIFOTI findings between an experienced clinician and a fifth-year dental student was high: $\kappa = 0.67$ for initial and $\kappa = 0.91$ for manifested carious lesions.	
Côrtes *et al* (2000)	To compare the performance of FOTI, visual inspection, and BW radiographs in the	*In vitro*	VE, BW, and DIFOTI	Occlusal	The reproducibilities of the FOTI, visual, and radiographic examinations were 0.87,	The radiographic method was poor at detecting lesions confined to enamel. FOTI, visual

(*Continued*)

Table 3.1. (*Continued*)

Author (year)	Aim	Protocol	Diagnostic tool(s)	Dental surface	Sensitivity/specificity/or statistical parameters	Main results/conclusions
	detection of occlusal caries and the estimation of lesion depth.				0.95, and 0.84, respectively (weighted kappa statistic). The intraexaminer reproducibility of the histological scores varied between 0.75 and 0.82 and the interexaminer reproducibility varied between 0.75 and 0.79. The consensus decision (by disagreement between examiners) was taken in less than 10% of the sample. For detection of lesions histologically extending into the dentin, the areas under the ROCs were 0.85, 0.83, and 0.87 for the FOTI, visual, and radiographic detection systems, respectively. No statistically significant differences were detected between the three methods.	inspection, and radiographs showed a good correlation with the histology but had difficulty in distinguishing lesions located deep in enamel or in the outer third of dentin. FOTI was shown to be as accurate as a detailed visual inspection in detecting occlusal caries.

Gomez *et al* (2013)	To appraise the performance of detection methods for NCCLs.	Systematic review	Visual, LF, or DD, radiographic, fiber-optic transillumination, and electrical conductance: (0.17–0.96), LF or DD (0.16–0.96), Radiographic (0.12–0.84), Fiber-optic transillumination (0.21–0.96), electrical conductance, and QLF	Not restricted	Sensitivity: visual: (0.17–0.96), LF or DD (0.16–0.96), radiographic (0.12–0.84), fiber-optic transillumination (0.21–0.96), electrical conductance (0.61–0.92), and QLF (0.82). Specificity: visual (0.46–1.0), LF or DD (0.25–1.00), radiographic (0.55–0.99), fiber-optic transillumination (0.74–0.88), electrical conductance (0.73–1.0), and QLF (0.92)	Visual methods should remain the standard for clinical assessment in dental practice. The diagnosis of NCCLs might be more accurately achieved by a combination of the visual method and other methods

enamel carious lesions. This study included optical coherence tomography, near-infrared, and FOTI/DiFOTI. Significant sensitivity differences were observed among the devices evaluated, in which a higher sensitivity was found for optical coherence tomography (0.94; 95% CI 0.88 to 0.97) compared to near-infrared (0.58; 95% CI 0.46 to 0.68) and FOTI/DIFOTI (0.47; 95% CI 0.35–0.59), but no significant difference was found for specificity. The authors observed that digital fiber-optic technologies present drawbacks in their capacity to detect enamel carious lesions, but may be considered to be consistent for the identification of sound teeth (Macey *et al* 2021). Also, in order to compile the data on this issue, a recent analysis of a systematic review assessed the diagnostic accuracies of technologies used to detect early caries in published Cochrane systematic reviews. The authors found a sensitivity of 0.76 (from 0.63 to 0.86) and a specificity of 0.82 (from 0.68 to 0.91) for transillumination methods. This review verified that the highest pairwise differences were noted in the summary sensitivity points for imaging and all other technologies but that the summary specificity points were generally similar. However, a low certainty of evidence was observed due to study limitations, inconsistency, and indirectness (Walsh *et al* 2022).

As for dentin caries, an *in vitro* study compared the performance of FOTI against those of visual inspection and bitewing radiographs for the detection of occlusal carious lesions; the lesion depth was also estimated for each tool. While the bitewing radiograph was shown to be a poor tool for the detection of lesions restricted to enamel (Côrtes *et al* 2003), FOTI, visual inspection, and radiographs demonstrated a strong correlation with histological findings, despite difficulties in distinguishing lesions located deep in enamel or in the outer third of dentin. In this study, the reproducibilities of FOTI, visual, and radiographic examinations were 0.87, 0.95, and 0.84, respectively (weighted kappa statistic) (Côrtes *et al* 2003). For the detection of lesions histologically extending into the dentin, the areas under the curve (AUCs) were 0.85, 0.83, and 0.87 for the FOTI, visual, and radiographic detection systems, respectively. No statistical difference was observed among the three methods evaluated. The authors concluded that FOTI was thus demonstrated to be as accurate as visual inspection for the detection of occlusal carious lesions.

In contrast with the abovementioned scenario observed under *in vitro* conditions, a systematic review observed that the performance of FOTI for dentin detection in occlusal carious lesions presented a sensitivity of 0.49 (ranging from 0.20 to 0.79), a specificity of 0.97 (ranging from 0.89 to 0.94), an AUC of 0.92, and a diagnostic odds ratio (DOR) of 37.77 (Kapor *et al* 2021). The authors stated, however, that the number of the included studies was too low and that further high-quality caries diagnostic studies would be required in order to provide sufficient data in relation to multiple caries thresholds. This trend was reported in a subsequent systematic review, which reported that further investigations will be necessary to reach more robust conclusions on this issue (Serban *et al* 2022).

Thus, despite the advantages of FOTI and DIFOTI, in light of the available evidence for the accuracy of these tools for caries diagnosis, both in enamel and dentin, regardless of the severity and surface location, it is reasonable to assume that more consistent evidence is still lacking, as the available reports do not reach a definitive conclusion, especially regarding the performance of illumination-based technologies on dentin tissue. In this sense, future studies with well-designed methodologies that better resemble *in vivo* conditions could help to strengthen the body of evidence on this subject.

3.4 Laser fluorescence

Among the physical methods used in the diagnosis of dental carious lesions in dentistry, fluorescence has been widely explored due to the incorporation of new instruments and technologies into the market. Laser fluorescence (example: DD pen) is a wavelength-based technology. A small laser produces excitation at a wavelength of 655 nm, resulting in red light. The DD pen is an instrument consisting of a display (example: DD display 2191) where values may be displayed, an integrated infrared diode, and an active tip pen (example: DD pen 2190) that emits excitation light and collects the resulting fluorescence. This tip may be exchanged for accessories (other tips) that better adapt to the surface of the tooth to be evaluated. The DD pen 2190 has a length of 220 mm, a diameter of 32 mm, a weight of 110 g, an infrared diode that operates at wavelengths from 850 nm to 950 nm, and a laser diode that operates at a wavelength of 655 nm. Due to the fact that a class one laser is used in this device, neither the professional nor the patient requires personal protective equipment (Abogazalah and Ando 2017, Pretty 2006).

A healthy tooth structure free of microbial biofilm produces little or no fluorescence. In the presence of a carious lesion, however, the tooth structure is altered and the metabolic activity present in the lesion favors changes in fluorescence. These changes are associated with protoporphyrin, a photosensitive pigment present in carious tissues (Abogazalah and Ando 2017, Pretty 2006).

Access to the product may be limited due to its high cost, which reached a figure of up to 3500 euros in 2022, but the application method is very practical. Laser fluorescence results in values that are presented in scores from zero to 99 in relation to the fluorescence degree detected in the dental tissue. Before starting to record the values, it is important to perform dental prophylaxis of the surfaces to prevent dirt from generating false positive results. The patient must also not have been submitted to the application of fluoride products prior to the exam, and the dental surfaces must be dry and free of saliva, considering that it may change the light direction. According to the manufacturer, when the evaluated tooth surfaces are pits or fissures, values of up to 12 indicate a healthy tooth structure, values from 13 to 24 indicate incipient demineralization, while values equal to or greater than 25 suggest intense demineralization. When the proximal surfaces of the teeth are evaluated, scores below seven indicate a structure without carious lesions, values from eight to 15 indicate the beginning of demineralization on the surface, and values above 16 indicate a structure with intense demineralization (Pretty 2006).

The effectiveness of laser fluorescence may be determined from its sensitivity and specificity in detecting carious lesions. Sensitivity is the probability that laser fluorescence will identify a dental caries lesion in a patient and that it is actually a true lesion; specificity, in turn, represents the probability that the test will identify the patient as healthy in situations in which there are effectively no carious lesions on the tooth structure. Good effectiveness is is denoted by high values of both parameters (Rosa *et al* 2016). A meta-analysis of cross-sectional studies that evaluated the degree of dental carious lesions in permanent teeth, comparing laser fluorescence and histological analysis, found that on occlusal surfaces the overall sensitivity and specificity values of the laser fluorescence method were 0.71 (0.69–0.73) and 0.81 (0.73–0.82), respectively. It was also observed that when a lesion increased in depth, the sensitivity of detection increased from 0.65 (0.59–0.70) in lesions restricted to enamel to 0.75 (0.72–0.78) in lesions that affected the inner half of the dentin. On the other hand, the test specificity was almost constant for different stages of the lesion (Rosa *et al* 2016).

A clinical study that evaluated 50 molars close to exfoliation in 24 children found that for early-stage occlusal lesions, visual/tactile inspection of the ICDAS index has the same degree of sensitivity and specificity as laser fluorescence, and the same behavior was observed for deep lesions involving dentin (Pontes *et al* 2017). *In vitro* studies of laser fluorescence also showed good diagnostic ability on occlusal surfaces (Serban *et al* 2022). For the diagnosis of proximal caries, a systematic review found that the sensitivity of laser fluorescence assessed *in vitro* and compared with histological assessments was 0.75 (0.62–0.90), while the specificity was 0.89 (0.76–0.95) (Janjic Rankovic *et al* 2021). Compared to visual inspection, superior results were found *in vivo* for laser fluorescence when separating the tooth or performing cavity preparation, achieving a sensitivity of 0.92 (0.82–0.96) and a specificity of 0.90 (0.73–0.97) (Janjic Rankovic *et al* 2021). Regarding the detection of secondary caries, laser fluorescence showed similar results to radiography in terms of the sensitivity and specificity parameters, achieving values of 0.50 (0.44–0.55) and 0.83 (0.78–0.88), respectively, and also presenting positive predictive values of 3.44 (2.53–4.70) and negative predictive values of 0.49 (0.34–0.70) (Brouwer *et al* 2016).

When interpreting the DD pen 2190 values, false positive results may be obtained if the following situations are not considered during the examination: the presence of dirt on the dental surfaces, composite resin restorations with fluorescent properties, dirty edges of composite resin restorations, dental calculus, areas close to the pulp (high values may be observed), food residues in pits and fissures, prophylactic paste residues, remineralized dental caries, strong natural fluorescence of the tooth structure, teeth with discolouration, and irradiated patients (radioactivity) (Abogazalah and Ando 2017, Pretty 2006).

In general, the available evidence indicates that laser fluorescence presents similar results to those obtained by traditional diagnostic methods for dental caries, such as visual examination and radiography, but these results need to be evaluated and interpreted with caution due to the high heterogeneity between studies and the scarcity of high-quality randomized clinical trials (Kapor *et al* 2021).

3.5 Quantitative light-induced fluorescence

Fluorescence results from light excitation of an object at a certain wavelength, and quantitative light-induced fluorescence (QLF) is based on a wavelength of 370 nm (in the blue region of the spectrum), which reaches the tooth structure. Enamel emits an autofluorescence that can be detected by an intraoral camera, producing an image composed predominantly of green (Pretty 2006). Autofluorescence is the result of light that passes through transparent enamel and excites fluorophores found at the enamel–dentin junction (Gomez 2015). A recent study revealed that the enamel autofluorescence observed using the QLF method is related to the enamel composition, particularly the inorganic–organic interface (Lee *et al* 2020). Fluorescence loss may be quantified relative to adjacent healthy tissue, assuming that healthy enamel represents 100% fluorescence. The image is recorded and digitized for quantification, and an area with a decrease in fluorescence greater than 5% is considered to represent demineralization of the tooth structure. In this case, the light is scattered back when it tries to cross carious lesions (Gomez 2015).

QLF™ technology is able to measure lesion area, depth, and volume as well as bacterial activity in terms of a percentage increase in red fluorescence. Red fluorescence is the result of bacterial metabolism (porphyrins), and there is a directly proportional relationship between its intensity and bacterial activity (Park *et al* 2022). The QLF equipment (Inspektor Dental Pro Quantitative Luz Care) cost approximately 1450 dollars in 2022 and consists of a light box containing a xenon lamp and a handpiece, plus a monitor that displays images and software (Gomez 2015).

A study of children evaluated the specificity and sensitivity of QLF in the detection of carious lesions on the occlusal and proximal surfaces of primary teeth at different stages of the lesion, comparing it with visual and tactile clinical examination (International Caries Detection and Assessment System II—ICDAS II) and with radiography (Cho *et al* 2021). Early (enamel without cavitation) or moderate (including enamel cavitation) dental carious lesions were used as criteria with which to assess the lesion stage. For early lesions of the occlusal surfaces, the method resulted in a mean sensitivity and specificity of 0.88 ± 0.83 and 0.82 ± 0.93, respectively, similar to the result obtained for moderate lesions, which achieved values of 0.90 ± 0.89 and 0.83 ± 0.76. On the other hand, in the proximal surface lesions, the mean sensitivity and specificity for early lesions were slightly lower, achieving values of 0.83 ± 0.73 and 0.74 ± 0.96, respectively. For moderate proximal surface lesions, the values of sensitivity and specificity were 0.91 ± 0.81 and 0.74 ± 0.91, respectively.

Comparing the data for the accuracy of QLF with laser fluorescence shows that both tests have similar levels of accuracy and do not show differences from the results achieved using visual examination (Pontes *et al* 2017). Thus, these technologies do not present obvious advantages over visual inspection of tooth structures in the diagnosis of occlusal carious lesions in primary teeth (Pontes *et al* 2017). For secondary caries detection, however, a meta-analysis showed that QLF is superior to the visual, tactile, radiographic, and laser fluorescence methods in terms of sensitivity but inferior in its specificity levels; the same analysis also highlighted positive predictive values of 1.70 (1.21–2.40) and negative predictive values of 0.57 (0.40–0.82) for QLF (Brouwer *et al* 2016).

The proposal to apply QLF in the diagnosis of dental carious lesions is interesting; however, the heterogeneity of the results and the scarcity of clinical studies mean that the results must be interpreted with caution. This directly affects clinical practice, as conventional methods (visual, tactile, and radiographic) remain the first-choice techniques for dental caries diagnosis (Brouwer *et al* 2016).

3.6 Cone beam computed tomography

In contrast with radiography-based methods, which provide two-dimensional images of three-dimensional structures, cone beam computed tomography (CBCT) is a tomography-based method in which the areas/structures of interest are seen through digital 'slices' obtained after scanning any given intraoral structures. Therefore, the issue of overlapping structures encountered in radiography-based methods is solved, which represents an improvement for the detection of incipient and secondary caries. Its main advantages include the use of a relatively low dose of radiation and greater efficiency for the detection of approximal lesions compared to interproximal radiography, as the results obtained using CBCT have greater sensitivity and lower specificity values (Kalathingal *et al* 2007, Aminoshariae *et al* 2018). In general, due to its high cost, CBCT is not widely used in daily clinical dental practice for the detection of dental caries. Instead, it is mainly used for the diagnosis and planning of surgical and/or endodontic procedures.

3.7 Conclusions

The body of evidence for complementary methods used for the detection of carious lesions attests their efficacy and safety for clinical use. The choice of any given method must take into account aspects such as cost, patient comfort, the compliance of uncooperative persons, the availability of equipment, the costs and expertise of the professional, and safety issues, especially for more vulnerable patients (e.g. children and pregnant women).

However, it must be emphasized that the efficacy of visual–tactile examination can be largely improved when basic procedures for clinical detection are followed (e.g. biofilm removal, dental drying, and light illumination), especially when standardized and validated methods, such as the International Caries Detection and Assessment System (ICDAS), are used. Other resources, including tooth separation, are simple, inexpensive, and extremely effective for the detection of proximal lesions. Therefore, auxiliary methods must only be used after thorough clinical examination, given that experienced professionals are often able to make their treatment decisions without the aid of complementary examination.

References and additional reading

Abogazalah N and Ando M 2017 Alternative methods to visual and radiographic examinations for approximal caries detection *J. Oral Sci.* **59** 315–22

Abogazalah N, Eckert G J and Ando M 2019 *In vitro* visual and visible light transillumination methods for detection of natural non-cavitated approximal caries *Clin. Oral Investig.* **23** 1287–294

Aminoshariae A, Kulild J C and Syed A 2018 Cone-beam computed tomography compared with intraoral radiographic lesions in endodontic outcome studies: a systematic review *J. Endod.* **44** 1626–631

Antipoviene A, Girijotaite M and Bendoraitiene E A 2020 Assessment of the depth of clinically detected approximal caries lesions using digital imaging fiber-optic transillumination in comparison to periapical radiographs *J. Oral Maxillofac. Res.* **11** e3

Antony D P, Thomas T and Nivedhitha M S 2020 Two-dimensional periapical, Panoramic radiography versus three-dimensional cone-beam computed tomography in the detection of periapical lesion after endodontic treatment: a systematic review *Cureus.* **12** 77–36

Basting R T and Serra M C 1999 Occlusal caries: diagnosis and noninvasive treatments *Quintessence Int.* **30** 174–8 https://www.quintpub.com/journals/qi/abstract.php?article_id=5320

Bourguignon C, Cohenca N and Lauridsen E *et al* 2020 International association of dental Traumatology guidelines for the management of traumatic dental injuries: 1. Fractures and luxations *Dent. Traumatol.* **36** 314–30

Braga M M, Mendes F M and Ekstrand K R 2010 Detection activity assessment and diagnosis of dental caries lesions *Dent. Clin. N. Am.* **54** 479–93

Brouwer F, Askar H, Paris S and Schwendicke F 2016 Detecting secondary caries lesions: a systematic review and meta-analysis *J. Dent. Res.* **95** 143–51

Brown C E Jr, Winkworth R J, Anderson O V and Jerman A C 1973 Degradation of dental radiographic processing solutions *J. Am. Dent. Assoc.* **87** 1200–5

Chauhan V and Wilkins R C 2019 A comprehensive review of the literature on the biological effects from dental X-ray exposures *Int. J. Radiat. Biol.* **95** 107–19 Epub 2019 Jan 24

Cho K H, Kang C M and Jung H I *et al* 2021 The diagnostic efficacy of quantitative light-induced fluorescence in detection of dental caries of primary teeth *J. Dent.* **115** 103845

Christie D A and Tansey E M (ed) 2006 *Development of Physics Applied to Medicine in the UK* (London: Wellcome Trust Centre for the History of Medicine) 1945–90 https://wellcomecollection.org/works/g6rqfsqh

Côrtes D F, Ellwood R P and Ekstrand K R 2003 An *in vitro* comparison of a combined FOTI/visual examination of occlusal caries with other caries diagnostic methods and the effect of stain on their diagnostic performance *Caries Res.* **37** 8–16

Dyson N A 1990 *X-Rays in Atomic and Nuclear Physics* 2nd edn (Cambridge: Cambridge University Press)

Evans R D 1955 *The Atomic Nucleus* (New York: McGraw-Hill)

Feynman R P, Leighton R B and Sands M 2006 *The Feynman Lectures in Physics* The New Millennium Edition (New York: Basic Books)

Foster Page L A, Boyd D and Fuge K *et al* 2018 The effect of bitewing radiography on estimates of dental caries experience among children differs according to their disease experience *BMC Oral Health* **18** 137

Gomez J, Tellez M, Pretty I A, Ellwood R P and Ismail A I 2013 Non-cavitated carious lesions detection methods: a systematic review *Community Dent. Oral. Epidemiol.* **41** 54–66

Gomez J 2015 Detection and diagnosis of the early caries lesion *BMC Oral Health* **15 Suppl 1** S3

Haak R, Wicht M J and Noack M J 2001 Conventional, digital and contrast-enhanced bitewing radiographs in the decision to restore approximal carious lesions *Caries Res.* **35** 193–9

Hardman P K, Tilmon M F and Taylor T S 1987 Radiographic solutions contamination *Oral Surg. Oral Med. Oral Pathol.* **63** 733–7

Hedin M 1989 Developing solutions for dental X-ray processors *Swed. Dent. J.* **13** 261–5

Hewitt P 2001 *Conceptual Physics* 9th edn (Toledo, OH: Addison-Wesley)

Hintze H, Wenzel A, Danielsen B and Nyvad B 1998 Reliability of visual examination, fibre-optic transillumination, and bite-wing radiography, and reproducibility of direct visual examination following tooth separation for the identification of cavitated carious lesions in contacting approximal surfaces *Caries Res.* **32** 204–9

Hubbell J H 2006 Review and history of photon cross section calculations *Phys. Med. Biol.* **51** 245–62

Janjic Rankovic M *et al* 2021 Systematic review and meta-analysis of diagnostic studies of proximal surface caries *Clin. Oral Investig.* **25** 6069–79

Kalathingal S M, Mol A, Tyndall D A and Caplan D J 2007 *In vitro* assessment of cone beam local computed tomography for proximal caries detection *Oral Surg. Oral Med. Oral Pathol. Oral Radiol. Endod.* **104** 699–704

Kapor S, Rankovic M J, Khazaei Y, Crispin A, Schüler I and Krause F *et al* 2021 Systematic review and meta-analysis of diagnostic methods for occlusal surface caries *Clin. Oral Investig.* **25** 4801–15

Kotzur I M 1994 W.C. Röntgen: a new type of ray *Radiology* **193** 329–32

Laitala M L, Piipari L, Sämpi N, Korhonen M, Pesonen P and Joensuu T *et al* 2017 Validity of digital imaging of fiber-optic transillumination in caries detection on proximal tooth surfaces *Int. J. Dent.* **2017** 8289636

Lee J Y, Kim H J, Lee E S, de Josselin de Jong E, Jung H I and Kim B I 2020 Quantitative light-induced fluorescence as a potential tool for detection of enamel chemical composition *Photodiagnosis Photodyn. Ther.* **32** 102054

Ludlow J B 1997 The efficacy of caries detection using three intraoral films under different processing conditions *J. Am. Dent.* **128** 1401–08

Macey R, Walsh T, Riley P, Hogan R, Glenny A M and Worthington H V *et al* 2021 Transillumination and optical coherence tomography for the detection and diagnosis of enamel caries *Cochrane Database Syst. Rev.* **1** CD013855

Machiulskiene V, Campus G, Carvalho J C, Dige I, Ekstrand K R and Jablonski-Momeni A *et al* 2020 Terminology of dental caries and dental caries management: consensus report of a workshop prganized by ORCA and cariology research group of IADR *Caries Res.* **54** 7–14

Marmaneu-Menero A, Iranzo-Cortés J E, Almerich-Torres T, Ortolá-Síscar J C, Montiel-Company J M and Almerich-Silla J M 2020 Diagnostic validity of digital imaging fiber-optic transillumination (DIFOTI) and near-infrared light transillumination (NILT) for caries in dentine *J. Clin. Med.* **9** 420

Murdoch-Kinch C A and McLean M E 2003 Minimally invasive dentistry *J. Am. Dent. Assoc.* **134** 87–95

Musri N, Christie B, Ichwan S J A and Cahyanto A 2021 Deep learning convolutional neural network algorithms for the early detection and diagnosis of dental caries on periapical radiographs: a systematic review *Imaging Sci. Dent.* **51** 237–42

Nair P N, Sjögren U, Figdor D and Sundqvist G 1999 Persistent periapical radiolucencies of root-filled human teeth, failed endodontic treatments, and periapical scars *Oral Surg. Oral Med. Oral Pathol. Oral Radiol. Endod.* **87** 617–27

Nyvad B, Machiulskiene V and Baelum V 1999 Reliability of a new caries diagnostic system Differentiating between active and inactive caries lesions *Caries Res.* **33** 252–60

Nyvad B 2004 Diagnosis versus detection of caries *Caries Res.* **38** 192–8

Park S, Lee E S, Jung H I and Kim B I 2022 Optical detection of oral biofilm in hospitalized geriatric patients using quantitative light-induced fluorescence technology *Photodiagnosis Photodyn. Ther* **39** 102962

Pitts N B, Zero D T, Marsh P D, Ekstrand K, Weintraub J A and Ramos-Gomez F *et al* 2017 Dental caries *Nat. Rev. Dis. Primers* **3** 17030

Pontes L R A, Novaes T F, Moro B L P, Braga M M and Mendes F M 2017 Clinical performance of fluorescence-based methods for detection of occlusal caries lesions in primary teeth *Braz. Oral Res.* **31** e91

Pontual A A, de Melo D P, de Almeida S M, Bóscolo F N and Haiter Neto F 2010 Comparison of digital systems and conventional dental film for the detection of approximal enamel caries *Dentomaxillofac. Radiol.* **39** 431–6

Pretty I A 2006 Caries detection and diagnosis: novel technologies *J. Dent.* **34** 727–39

Ricketts D N, Ekstrand K R, Martignon S, Ellwood R, Alatsaris M and Nugent Z 2007 Accuracy and reproducibility of conventional radiographic assessment and subtraction radiography in detecting demineralization in occlusal surfaces *Caries Res.* **41** 121–8

Rosa M I, Schambeck V S, Dondossola E R, Alexandre M C, Tuon L and Grande A J *et al* 2016 Laser fluorescence of caries detection in permanent teeth *in vitro*: a systematic review and meta-analysis *J. Evid. Based Med.* **9** 213–24

Schneiderman A, Elbaum M, Shultz T, Keem S, Greenebaum M and Driller J 1997 Assessment of dental caries with digital imaging fiber-optic transillumination (DIFOTI): *in vitro* study *Caries Res.* **31** 103–10

Serban C, Lungeanu D, Bota S D, Cotca C C, Negrutiu M L and Duma V F *et al* 2022 Emerging technologies for dentin caries detection—a systematic review and meta-analysis *J. Clin. Med.* **11** 674

Sharan R, Thankappan K and Iyer S *et al* 2011 Intraoperative transillumination to determine the extent of frontal sinus in subcranial approach to anterior skull base *Skull Base* **21** 71–4

Simón-Soro A and Mira A 2015 Solving the etiology of dental caries *Trends Microbiol* **23** 76–82

Röntgen W C 1896 On a new kind of rays *Nature* **53** 274–76 Translated by Arthur Stanton from the Sitzungsberichte der Würzburger Physic-Medic. Gesellschaft

Strassler H E and Pitel M L 2014 Using fiber-optic transillumination as a diagnostic aid in dental practice *Compend. Contin. Educ. Dent.* **35** 80–8

Struzycka I 2014 The oral microbiome in dental caries *Pol. J. Microbiol.* **63** 127–35

Tagliaferro E, Junior A V, Rosell F L, Silva S, Riley J L and Gilbert G H *et al* 2019 Caries diagnosis in dental practices: results from dentists in a brazilian community *Oper. Dent.* **44** E23–31

Tinanoff N, Baez R J, Diaz Guillory C, Donly K J, Feldens C A and McGrath C *et al* 2019 Early childhood caries epidemiology, aetiology, risk assessment, societal burden, management, education, and policy: global perspective *Int. J. Paediatr. Dent.* **29** 238–48

Turner J E 2004 Interaction of ionizing radiation with matter *Health Phys.* **86** 228–52

Vijayan A K, Jo S, Mathew B, Vidyadharan M and Nair A M 2022 Comparison of diagnostic ability of conventional film and storage phosphor plate in detecting proximal caries with direct measurements by stereomicroscope: a diagnostic test evaluation *Contemp. Clin. Dent.* **13** 156–61

Walsh T, Macey R, Ricketts D, Carrasco Labra A, Worthington H and Sutton A J *et al* 2022 Enamel caries detection and diagnosis: an analysis of systematic reviews *J. Dent. Res.* **101** 261–69

Webb S 1990 *From the Watching of Shadows: The Origins of Radiological Tomography* 1st edn (Boca Raton, FL: CRC Press)

Wenzel A and Møystad A 2010 Work flow with digital intraoral radiography: a systematic review *Acta Odontol. Scand.* **68** 106–14

Wenzel A 2004 Bitewing and digital bitewing radiography for detection of caries lesions *J. Dent. Res.* **83** 72–5

Wenzel A 2021 Radiographic modalities for diagnosis of caries in a historical perspective: from film to machine-intelligence supported systems *Dentomaxillofac. Radiol* **50** 20210010

White S C and Pharoah M J 2004 X-ray film, intensifying screens, and grids *Oral Radiology Principles and Interpretation* 5 (St Louis, MO: Mosby) p 744

Young H 1999 *University Physics* (Reading, MA: Addison-Wesley)

Chapter 4

Cone beam computed tomography: a diagnostic innovation in dentistry

Manisha M Khorate and Aniket Vaidya

Since the invention of conventional computed tomography (CT) in 1967 by Sir Godfrey Hounsfield, three-dimensional imaging has evolved gradually. Cone beam computed tomography (CBCT), a relatively advanced imaging modality, has been widely used in the last decade because of its multiple applications in dentomaxillofacial diagnosis.

The clinical applications of CBCT include the evaluation of hard tissue, implant planning, determination of the extents of tumors/cysts, demonstrations of root canal anatomy, etc. In addition to its use in dentistry, CBCT can be applied in assessing craniofacial traumas, oropharyngeal volumes, and the ear, nose, and throat (ENT) regions. CBCT provides higher quality 3D imaging and overcomes the disadvantages of conventional radiography, namely radiation exposure, image distortion, and cost.

The aims of this chapter are to acquaint physicists with the operational principles of CBCT and highlight its advantages with respect to the image reproducibility and quality of this novel technique. It further focuses on the diagnostic, treatment planning, and prognostic applications of CBCT in maxillofacial as well as head and neck imaging.

4.1 Introduction

CBCT offers three-dimensional visualization and more accurate imaging compared to analog and digital radiographs. Since its inception, it has attracted unprecedented interest from all fields of dentistry as well as the medical field. It is an accurate tool for many clinical oral–maxillofacial indications and uses lower radiation doses than those of computed tomography (CT). Conventional CT uses a fan-shaped x-ray beam that rotates in a helical fashion around the patient; the data is acquired by solid-state detectors located around the gantry (figure 4.1). The images obtained are

doi:10.1088/978-0-7503-5316-8ch4

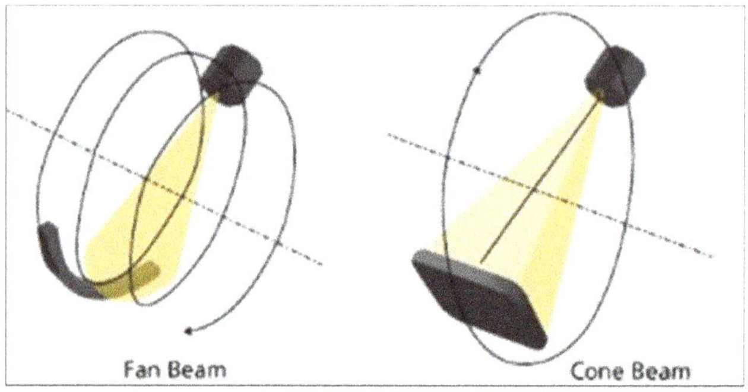

Figure 4.1. The shape of the x-ray beam in CT (fan beam) versus CBCT (cone beam).

typically 'axial' cross sections through the region of interest (ROI), but computer algorithm reformatting enables us to view the ROI in the coronal and sagittal planes along with 3D reconstructions. In contrast, CBCT scanners use a cone-shaped beam of x-rays that rotates around the object of interest to produce a volume of data; it uses a two-dimensional extended digital array as an areal detector (figure 4.1). The clinician must determine the risk:benefit ratio with regards to Imaging and the selection of patient. Clinicians worldwide are rapidly realizing the significant benefits of CBCT imaging. This chapter presents an overview of CBCT imaging.

4.2 The fundamentals of cone beam CT technology

An in-depth discussion of the physics of CBCT technology is beyond the scope of this text. This section focuses on the key fundamentals of the CBCT principle. The CBCT radiation source consists of a conventional low-radiation x-ray tube. The resultant cone-shaped beam is projected onto a flat-panel detector (FPD) or a charge-coupled device (CCD) with an image intensifier [1]. The cone-shaped beam used in CBCT produces a more focused beam which is responsible for much less radiation scatter than the fan shapes of conventional CT devices (figure 4.1) [2]. As a result, the total absorbed radiation due to CBCT is approximately 20% of the total absorbed radiation due to conventional CT [3].

4.2.1 Image acquisition

The tube and the detector perform a single rotation of either 180° or 360° around the patient. The cone beam is targeted at the selected region. In this technique, the x-ray source and reciprocating area detector synchronously move around the patient's head, which is stabilized with a head holder. Multiple exposures are taken at fixed intervals (angles) during the single rotational scan without the need for patient movement. Each of these exposures is referred to as a basis image or projection [1, 3]. Once the scan is complete and all the basis images are made, the complete set of basis images forms the 'projection data' [3]. The total number of basis images depends upon the choice of voxel size and the scanner's capability. The selection of the smallest voxel size results in a greater number of basis images, a longer scan time, a greater radiation dose, and better-quality constructed images. Software algorithms are used to reconstruct the slice data or basis images, which can then be viewed in user-defined planes i.e. axial, sagittal, or coronal.

4.2.2 The field of view

The size of the scanned object volume is called the field of view (FOV). For units with a flat-panel detector, the FOV is a cylindrical shape in the center of the scanner between the detector and the x-ray source. The manufacturers of the CBCT machine ensure that the machine is programmed to scan FOVs of various sizes and areas [3]. The range of commercially available FOVs for flat-panel detectors is summarized in table 4.1. In contrast to conventional CT, the CBCT unit provides the operator with the flexibility of reducing the FOV to the ROI. This is in accordance with the 'as low as reasonably achievable' (ALARA) principle because of the ability of the CBCT unit to focus the beam on the ROI and cause minimal residual scatter to the surrounding tissues. Thus, it is recommended to limit the FOV size to the smallest volume that can accommodate the ROI (figure 4.2).

Table 4.1. The ranges of FOVs of commercially available CBCT units.

No.	Model	FOVs (in cms)	Software
1.	*Planmeca ProMax 3D Mid (Planmeca)*	*4 × 5, 4 × 8, 8 × 5, 8 × 8, 10 × 6, 16 × 6, 10 × 10, 16 × 10, 16 × 17, 20 × 6, 20 x 10, 20 × 17*	*Romexis*
2.	*Axeos (Dentsply Sirona)*	*5 × 5.5, 8 × 8, 11 × 10, 17 × 13*	*Sidexis*
3.	*i-CAT*	*8 × 8, 16 × 4, 16 × 6, 16 × 8, 16 × 10, 16 × 11, 23 x 17*	*Tx STUDIO*
4.	*CS 9600 (Carestream Dental)*	*4 × 4, 5 × 5, 6 × 6, 5 × 8, 8 × 5, 10 × 5, 12 × 5, 8 × 8, 10 × 10, 12 × 10, 16 × 6, 16 × 10*	*CS imaging software*
5.	*GiANO HR (Newtom)*	*6 × 6, 8 × 6, 8 × 8, 10 × 6, 10 × 8, 10 × 10, 13 x 8, 13 x 10, 13 × 14, 13 × 16, 15 × 6, 16 × 10, 16 × 18*	*NNT Software*

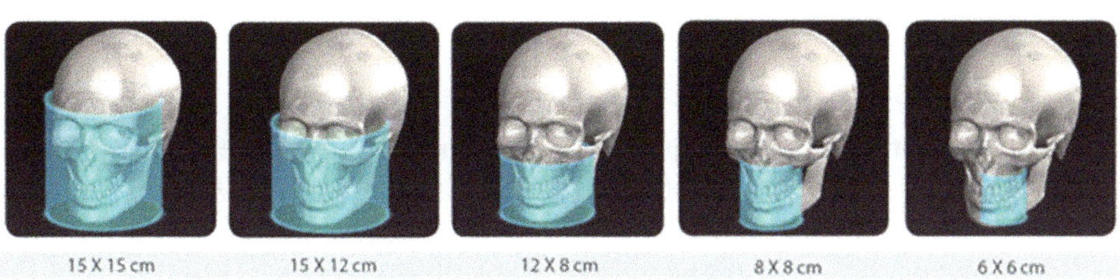

Figure 4.2. FOVs of various sizes and areas.

4.2.3 Voxels

A 'VOlume piXEL,' or voxel, represents the smallest distinguishable cuboid of a 3D image; it is similar to the pixel representation used for 2D data [4]. A 'picture element,' or pixel, is a small rectangle whose size ranges between 20 and 60 microns. However, the 'pixel' in a CBCT machine is a 'voxel' or volume element. It is basically a cube, i.e. each of its sides has has the same length. In conventional medical CT, the pixel is 'non-isotropic'; it has two equal sides but the third, or '*z*'-plane, has a selectable width that can range in size from 1.0 mm to 1.0 cm or more. Although CT voxel surfaces can be as small as 0.625 mm square, their depth is usually on the order of 1–2 mm. In CBCT, each side of an isotropic voxel has the same length or dimensions. This results in submillimeter resolutions ranging from 0.4 mm to as low as 0.125 mm.

4.2.4 Gray scale

The ability of a CBCT scan to display differences in attenuation is called gray scale. The units used for this parameter are bits, and the number of bits determines the number of shades of gray available to display the attenuation. Most current CBCT machines have 12–16 bit detectors and are capable of identifying 4096–65 536 shades of gray.

4.2.5 Radiation exposure

Radiology is an indispensable tool in dentistry. Its value in treatment planning, monitoring disease progression, and assessing treatment outcome cannot be emphasized enough. However, the use of radiology introduces the risk of exposure for patients and clinical staff. Most medical imaging is used less often than the frequency with which dentists use radiology. This is due to the use of intraoral radiography, which is readily available at the chairside. The effective radiation doses for CBCT are typically far less than the levels used in clinical spiral CT. The reported radiation dose levels vary according to the CBCT device being assessed, from around 10 μSv to 1200 μSv, which is the equivalent of 2–240 panoramic radiographs [5]. Another study found that the absorbed x-ray dose due to CBCT ranged from 40 to 500 μSv depending upon the machine and volume size [6]. The operator must remember that even for the same machine, there can be a huge variation in the effective dosage because of variable options such as multiple FOVs and exposure settings.

4.3 The advantages of CBCT

- **Dose reduction:** published data for CBCT indicate that the effective radiation dose is between 0.035 and 0.10 mSv. This is almost 80%–90% less than the dose caused by conventional CT (the effective dose for CT of the mandible and maxilla being 0.4 mSv – Newcastle University Trust Hospitals data [4]).
- **X-ray beam limitation:** reducing the size of the irradiated area by limiting the FOV to the ROI significantly minimizes the radiation dose.

- **Rapid scan times:** all the basis images or projections are acquired in a single rotation; thus, the scan time is short, varying between 10 and 40 s. Fast scan times also eliminate artifacts due to patient movement.
- **Image accuracy:** isotropic voxels capable of producing submillimetre resolutions increase the accuracy of scans.
- **Artifact Reduction:** in CT scans of the oral region, the presence of metallic dental restorations causes a problem due to streak artifacts, which can significantly reduce the diagnostic quality of the image. CBCT imaging also produces streak artifacts due to metal restorations but artifact removal algorithms provide superior quality images of the dental structures (see section 4.6).
- **Volume Manipulation:** the ability of the CBCT software to realign the viewing plane with the long axis of any tooth provides the observer with an appropriate angle at which to interpret the local anatomy.

4.4 The limitations of CBCT

- The inherent limitations of CBCT limit the use of this technology, and in some circumstances, other modes of imaging have proved to be more beneficial. For example, caries detection and the evaluation of teeth with dense metal prosthetic restorations are not performed well by CBCT due to beam hardening artifacts. Intraoral analog and digital radiography are the preferred modalities in such cases.
- CBCT does not show any soft-tissue detail.
- Motion artifacts are seen due to the long scan times. This drawback is addressed in newer machines by quicker scan times and improved patient head positioning and stabilizing devices.

4.5 Applications

4.5.1 Implantology

The chances of successful implant placement increase when the available edentulous alveolar ridge is adequate in width and height for an even distribution of masticatory forces. For implant treatment planning, it is important to evaluate the planned bone site both quantitatively and qualitatively. The radiologist should be able to assess the vital anatomic structures around the implant site. By careful evaluation, the need for bone grafting or augmentation procedures can be planned simultaneously. The ability to produce cross-sectional images along curved maxillas or mandibles has rendered CBCT an ideal tool for dental implant planning. Para-axial slices that have a thickness of 0.1–0.2 mm at 1–2 mm intervals provide the most accurate cross-sectional images. Accurate measurements of bone height and width are essential to implant size selection. Along with the width and height measurements, the ridge morphology can be assessed in the buccolingual plane, which is otherwise impossible in two-dimensional radiology. The most commonly encountered alveolar ridge shapes are rectangular, pyramidal, and hourglass shapes (figures 4.3–4.6). The angulation of the ridge needs to be checked in order to plan the implant insertion path.

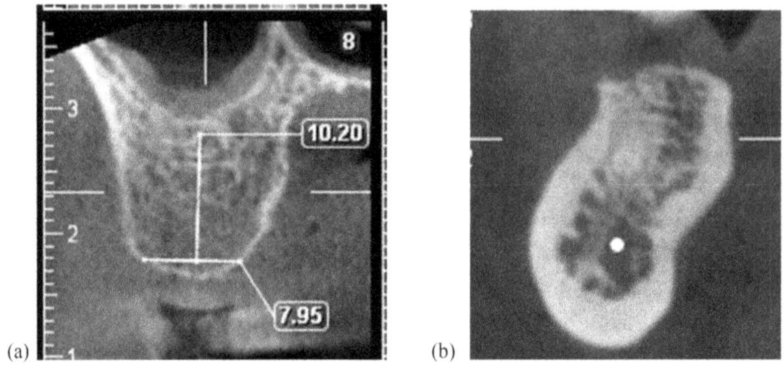

Figure 4.3. (a) Rectangular-type alveolar ridge morphology in the maxillary posterior segment. (b) Rectangular-type alveolar ridge morphology in the mandibular posterior region.

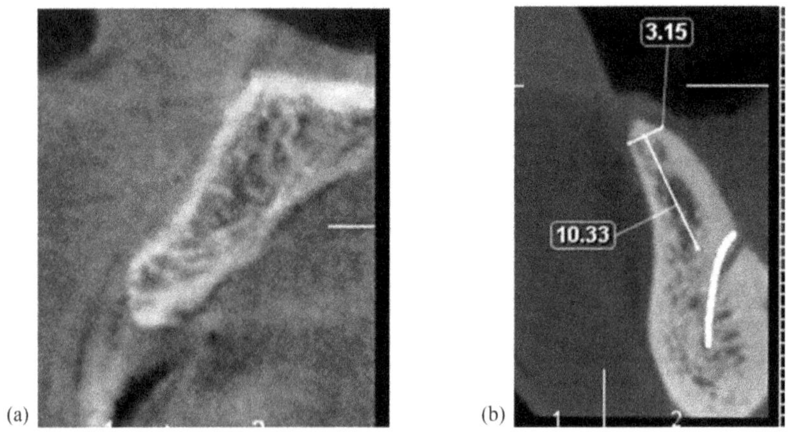

Figure 4.4. (a) A pyramidal-shaped alveolar ridge morphology in the maxillary anterior region. (b) A pyramidal-shaped alveolar ridge morphology in the mandibular anterior region along with nerve marking for nerve canal incision.

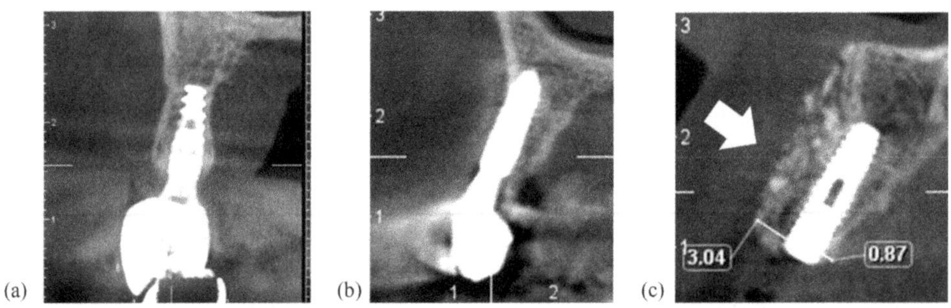

Figure 4.5. (a) A hourglass-shaped alveolar ridge morphology in the maxillary premolar region. One should exercise caution before planning an implant in this region due to the risk of perforation. (b) A hourglass-shaped alveolar ridge morphology in the maxillary premolar region in which the implant is seen engaging with the buccal cortical bone. (c) Augmenting the buccal portion of an hourglass-shaped alveolar ridge with a bone graft (white arrow).

Bone measurements: As a rule of thumb, a distance of 1.5 mm is maintained between an implant and the vital structures and minimum distances of 2 mm and 3 mm are maintained from adjacent teeth and adjacent implants, respectively. For the maxillary anterior region, the available bone height is measured from the crest of the ridge to the floor of the nasal cavity. In the maxillary posterior region, the height is measured from the crest of the alveolar ridge to the floor of the maxillary sinus. In the mandibular anterior region, the bone height is measured from the crest of the ridge to the inferior border of the mandible, and in the mandibular posterior region, it is measured from the crest of the ridge to the superior cortex of the inferior alveolar nerve canal (figures 4.7 and 4.8).

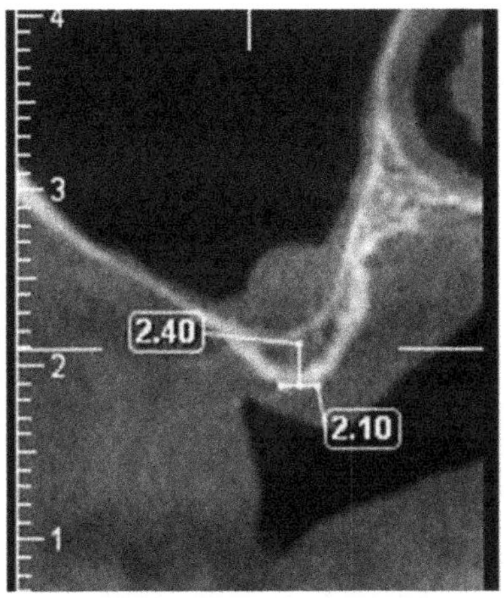

Figure 4.6. An extremely resorbed maxillary alveolar ridge with a minimal soft-tissue density shadow over the floor of the maxillary sinus.

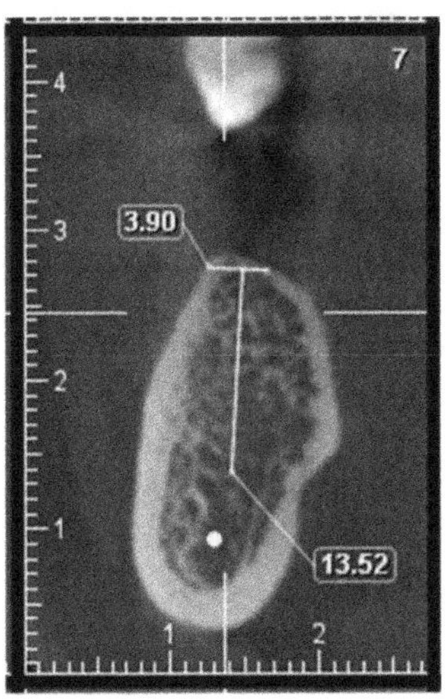

Figure 4.7. A measurement of bone height in the mandibular posterior region.

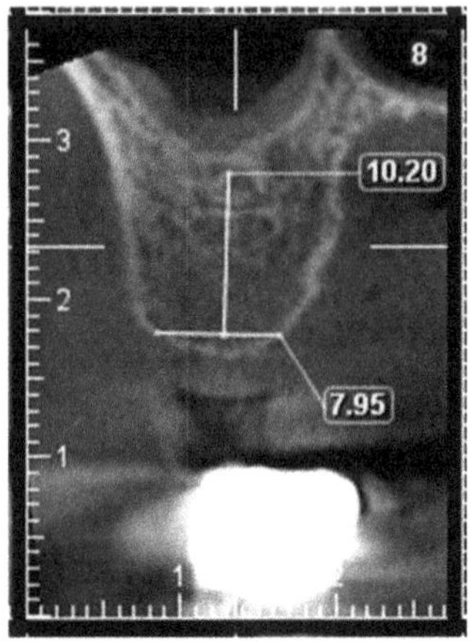

Figure 4.8. A measurement of bone height in the maxillary posterior region.

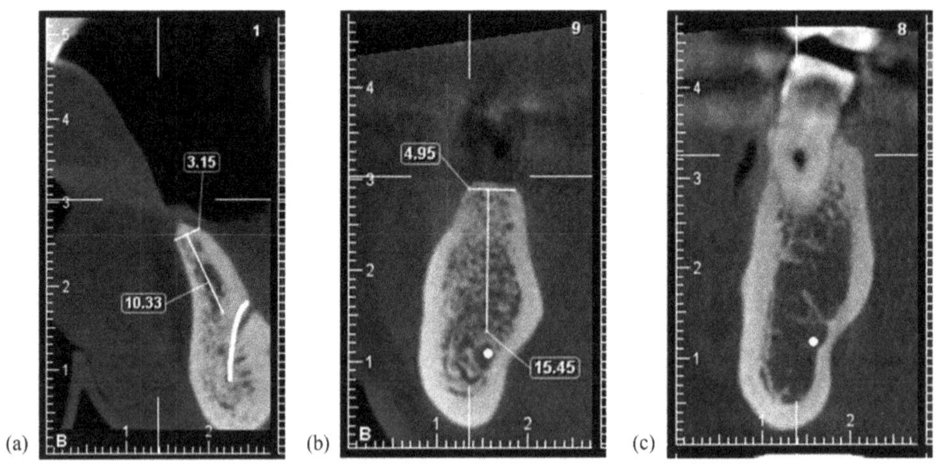

Figure 4.9. (a) Homogenous cortical bone. (b) Thin cortical bone with dense trabeculae of good quality. (c) Thin cortical bone with very low-density trabeculae.

Bone quality: the voxel values obtained in CBCT are not absolute values, unlike the Hounsfield units (HUs) used in CT. HUs provide a quantitative assessment of bone density. At present, to the best knowledge of the authors, there is no standard system for scaling gray scales in reconstructed CBCT images.

Bone quality can be subjectively classified into the following groups (figure 4.9):

I. Homogenous cortical bone
II. Thick cortical bone with a marrow cavity
III. Thin cortical bone with dense trabeculae of good quality
IV. Very thin cortical bone with low-density trabeculae

Virtual implant planning: numerous manufacturer-provided and third-party software suites are available with interactive interfaces that simulate implant placement at edentulous sites. Such software considers the shape, size, and spatial orientation of the planned implant. It also allows for proper abutment selection. Realistic implant images can be viewed and moved in space so that the most appropriate insertion path is selected (figures 4.10–4.12). Key points to remember for successful implant planning are as follows:

- Maintain a distance of 1–1.5 mm on either side of the implant fixture.
- Maintain a distance of 1–2 mm between the base of the implant and any adjacent anatomic structures (for example, the sinus floor or nerve canal).
- Determine the type of buccolingual ridge morphology.
- Determine the ridge angulation with respect to the vertical plane.
- Occlusal forces acting on the implant fixture should be parallel or almost parallel to the vertical axis of the alveolar ridge.

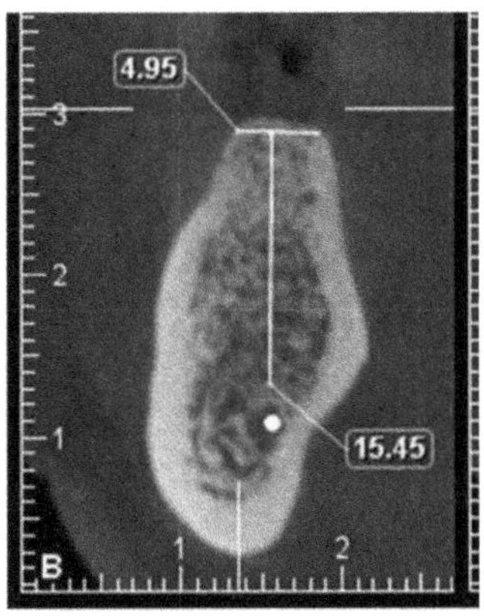

Figure 4.10. Bone height measurements maintaining a distance of at least 2 mm from the inferior alveolar nerve canal

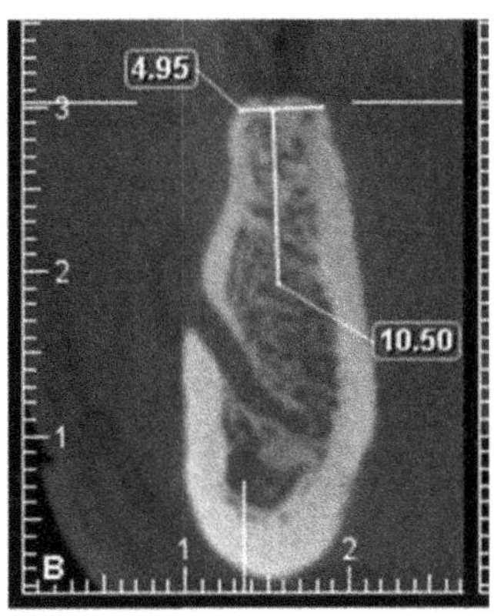

Figure 4.11. Bone height measurements in the region of the mental foramen opening in the mandibular alveolar ridge

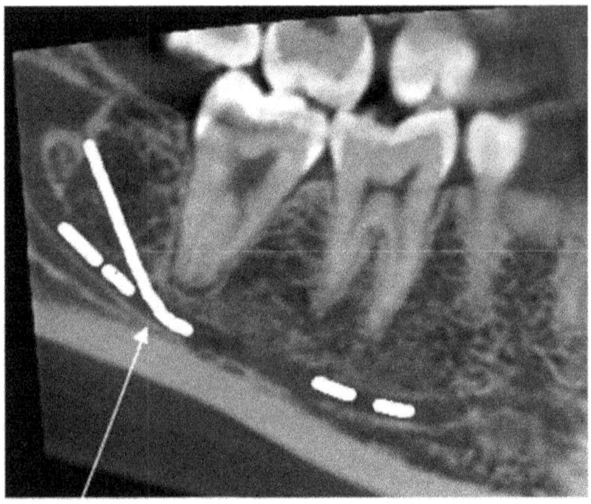

Figure 4.12. A sagittal section showing presence of the bifid inferior alveolar nerve canal. Such anatomic variations are uncommon, but whenever present they have to be taken into consideration during implant planning.

4.5.2 Periodontology

Periodontitis is an extremely common disease in which there is inflammation of the tissue around the teeth, often causing recession of the gingiva and loosening of the teeth. Two-dimensional intraoral radiography is routinely employed to investigate periodontal findings and alveolar bone loss. However, it has a limited role in diagnosing buccal and lingual bone defects. The ability to visualize the alveolar bone in three dimensions significantly improves periodontal diagnosis. CBCT is superior in diagnosing buccal and lingual defects as well as evaluating the involvement of furcation in multirooted teeth. CBCT provides substantial information about root morphology and is more effective in diagnosing bony fenestration and dehiscence. When a guided tissue regeneration (GTR) membrane is placed in an interproximal area, adjusting the membrane according to the anatomy of the roots and bone defects is time consuming and prolongs the surgery. Based on information provided by CBCT images, the GTR membrane can be precut into the desired shape, thus shortening the intraoperative time spent adjusting the GTR membrane.

Illustrative case 01: Maxillary Sinusitis secondary to Oro-antral, communication

A 70-year-old male patient reported with a complaint of pain and heaviness on the right side of his face. A clinical examination revealed gingival recession and mobility of the right maxillary first molar. A 2D panoramic radiograph showed severe alveolar bone loss in relation to the right upper first molar, which was suggestive of severe localized periodontitis. A CBCT scan revealed periapical bone loss along with perforation of the floor of the maxillary sinus and a soft-tissue density shadow in the floor of the maxillary sinus suggestive of reactionary sinusitis. CBCT revealed the cause of the alveolar bone loss to be a fracture of the mesiobuccal root of the first molar (figure case 4.1).

(a)
(b)
(c)

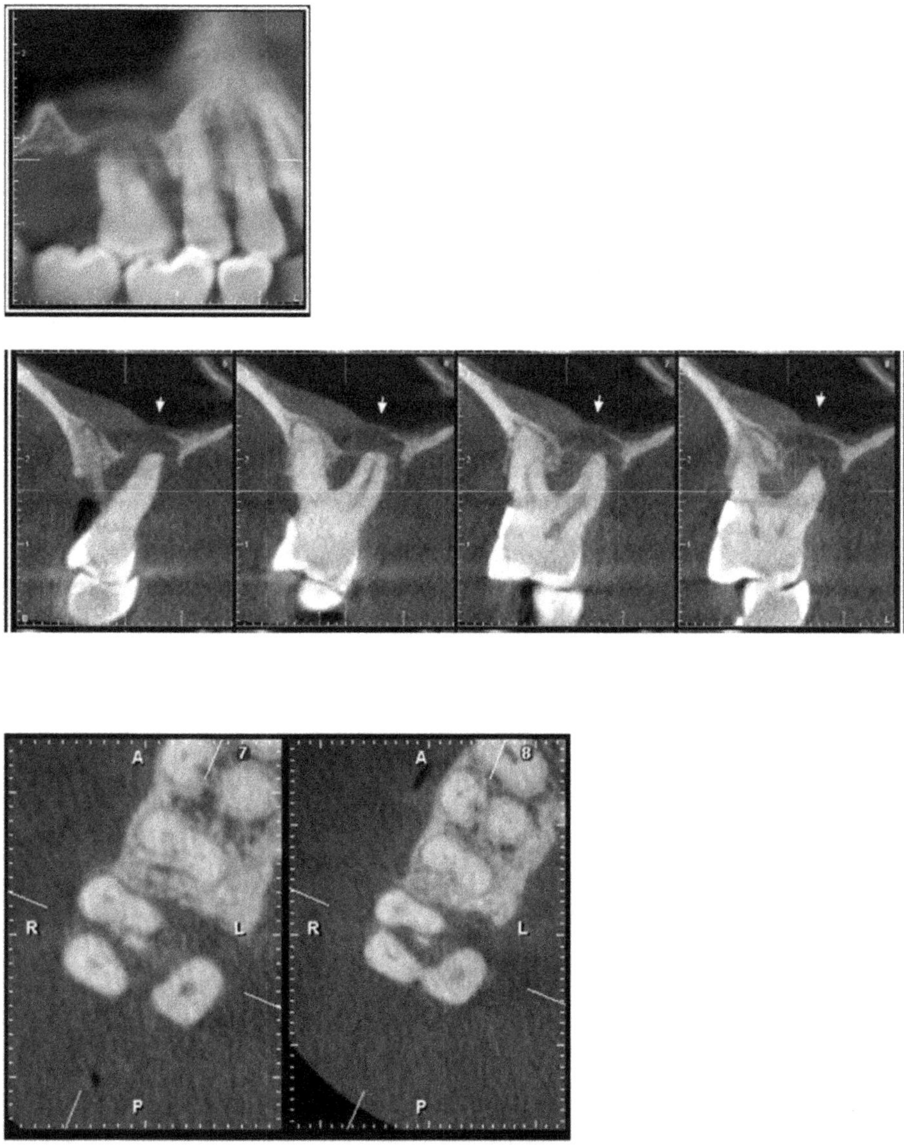

Figure case 4.1. (a) A cropped panoramic view. (b) Sagittal sections at 1 mm intervals showing the presence of oro-antral communication along with mild maxillary sinusitis. (c) Axial sections showing a fracture of a portion of the mesiobuccal root. The radiographic differential diagnosis may be cemental tears.

4.5.3 Endodontics

In endodontics, CBCT is useful in the assessment of accessory root canals, anatomical variations of the canals, the presence of periapical pathology, periradicular surgical planning, and dentoalveolar trauma evaluation. It is used for evaluating the borders of periapical pathologies without the superimposition of adjacent structures. It is particularly useful in checking the occurrence of periapical lesions associated with the individual roots of molars. In one study, CBCT was suggested to be superior to periapical radiographs in the characterization of periapical radiolucent lesions, reliably demonstrating lesion proximity to the maxillary sinus, sinus membrane involvement, and the lesion location relative to the mandibular canal [7]. CBCT also demonstrated superiority to 2D radiographs in detecting vertical and horizontal fractured roots and whether they are buccolingual or mesiodistal. The C-shaped canal variation presents a challenge to endodontists who perform root canal surgery. It is easy to distinguish the C-shaped canal anatomy in CBCT, which helps endodontists to locate the canal and prevent instrumentation mishaps. In maxillary molars, the MB2 canal is readily revealed in CBCT (figures 4.13–4.17).

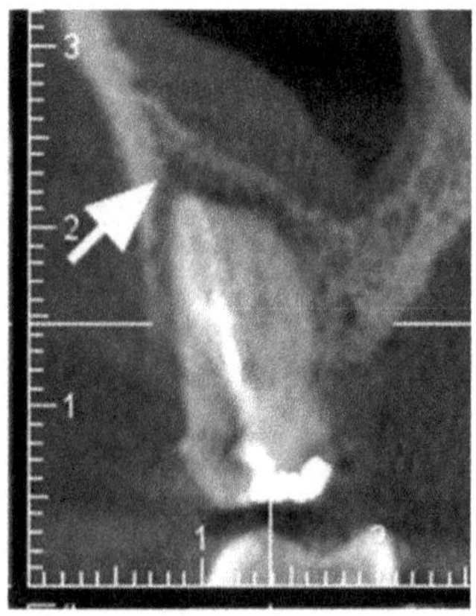

Figure 4.13. A coronal section through the maxillary premolar showing periradicular hypodensity (loss of alveolar bone) suggestive of a periapical abscess.

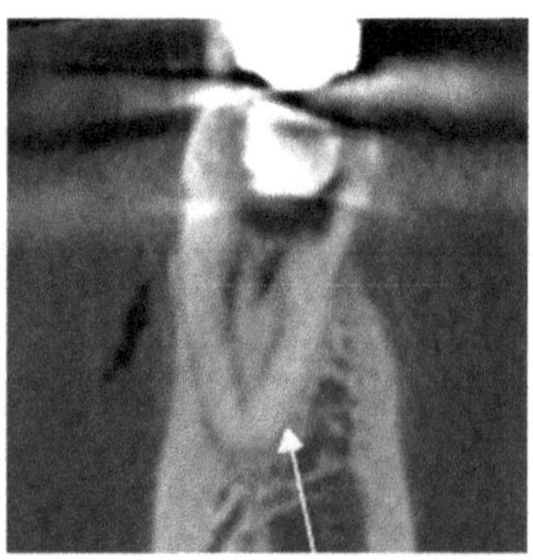

Figure 4.14. Vertucci's type II root canal configuration [8] in the mandibular second molar.

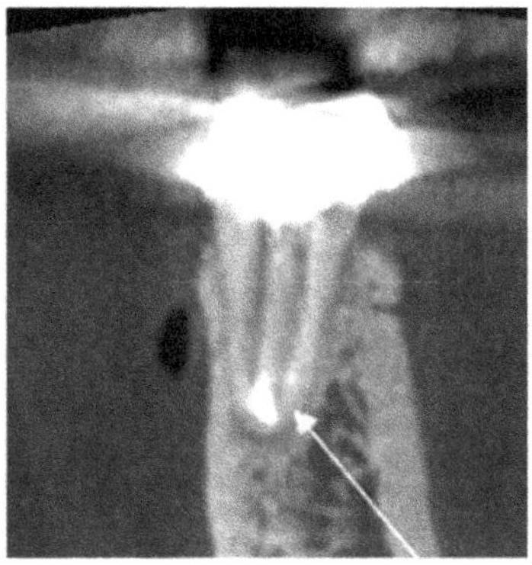

Figure 4.15. Vertucci's type IV root canal configuration (F. J. Vertucci 1984) in the mandibular first molar.

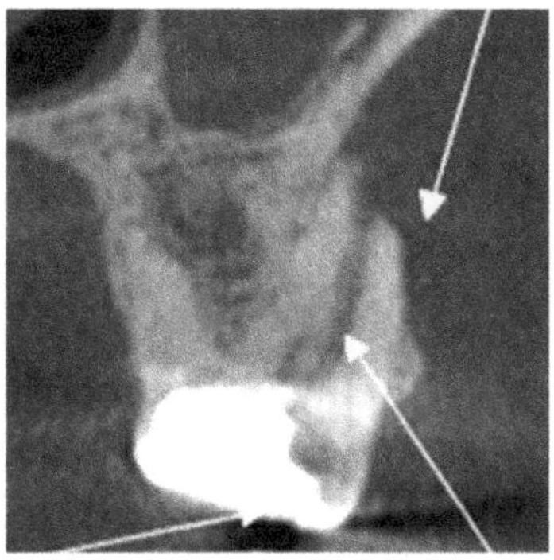

Figure 4.16. External root resorption of the mesiobuccal root of the maxillary first molar.

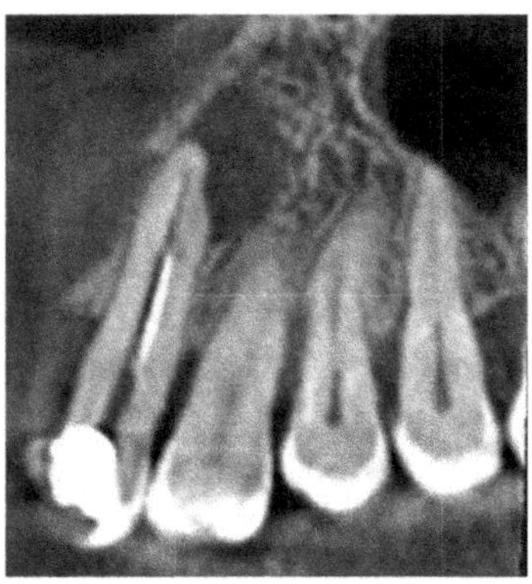

Figure 4.17. An oblique sagittal section showing inadequate obturation of the lateral incisor, the presence of a radicular cyst, and external root resorption.

4.5.4 Orthodontics

The most recognized and accepted use for CBCT in orthodontics is for the evaluation of impacted teeth, especially the canines. The tube-shift method is traditionally used for evaluating the labial or palatal position of an impacted canine. This method provides an arbitrary position of the impacted tooth. CBCT imaging not only helps in precisely locating the position of the impacted tooth but also displays the exact angulation and orientation of the impacted tooth. The temporary anchorage device (TAD) has recently gained popularity in orthodontics. Tooth movements are easily accomplished using TAD anchorage. Knowledge of the root position is essential for successful placement of a TAD. CBCT images allow accurate and dependable views of the root positions and the interradicular space as compared to panoramic or intraoral views. The quality and density of alveolar bone at the proposed site of TAD insertion can also be assessed using CBCT.

4.5.5 Craniofacial trauma

Recently, CBCT has increasingly been used to evaluate craniofacial fractures. The first case report on the use of CBCT was published in 2000 [9]. After that, several case reports and studies involving the use of CBCT for craniofacial trauma have come to light. Since CBCT is a low-dose, high-resolution imaging modality, is preferred in cases of mandibular and orbital floor fractures. It is important to point out that although CBCT can demonstrate orbital content herniation in orbital floor fractures, the lack of soft-tissue contrast falls short of differentiating the tissue compositions of the herniated materials. In cases in which tooth fractures are suspected, it may be difficult to take intraoral radiographs immediately post-trauma because of bleeding, swelling, and patient discomfort. In addition, in order to spot a fracture line on a tooth, or, in other words, to identify a radiolucent fracture line on the image, it is essential that the x-rays pass through the gap of the fracture. To accomplish this, several intraoral views are required at different angulations. In such cases, a CBCT scan can be quickly acquired and the teeth can be viewed from all angles to diagnose fracture lines. CBCT is also useful in helping dentists to understand the postoperative statuses of patients with maxillofacial fractures (figures 4.18 and 4.19).

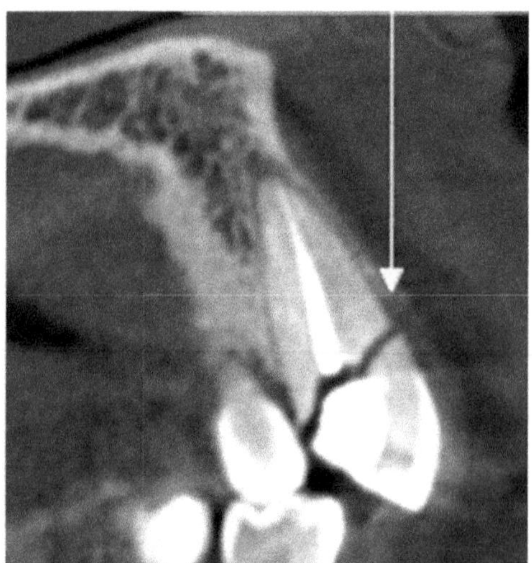

Figure 4.18. An oblique sagittal section showing a horizontal fracture in the cervical third of the root.

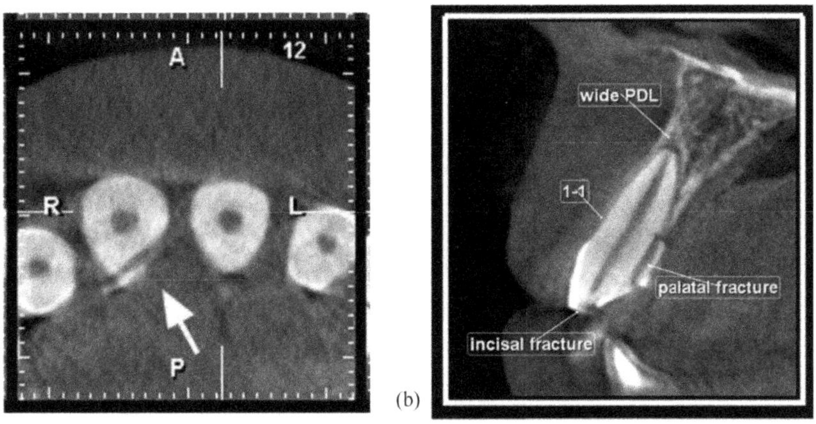

(a) (b)

Figure 4.19. (a) Axial sections through a maxillary central incisor in a patient with a history of trauma to the face, showing a fracture of the palatal portion of the root. (b) An oblique sagittal view of the same tooth showing the vertical fracture on the palatal surface of the root. This was undiagnosed by clinical examination and 2D intraoral radiography.

4.5.6 Temporomandibular joint (TMJ) morphology

A panoramic view is an acceptable initial tool with which to screen the TMJ morphology. However, because of superimpositions the osseous details of the TMJ may be obscured to the observer. CBCT images of the TMJ can produce slices at 1–2 mm intervals and hence can better demonstrate the morphology of condyles. The higher resolution of CBCT permits the detection of condylar erosions with greater reliability as compared to that of CT. In the TMJ, the presence of erosions and osteophytes is a radiographic clue that an active degenerative process may be occurring. Erosions are radiographically defined as a local area in the condyle with decreased density in the cortical joint surface. Adaptive changes are also sometimes evident in the form of subcortical bone sclerosis. To be able to clearly identify the presence of erosions and osteophytes, an unobstructed view of the joint and surrounding structures is required [10]. CBCT images are far superior in detecting surface erosions over the condyle as well as the presence of osteophytes. In CBCT, coronal views are of high image quality and give information about the pathological processes which is not seen in the views. In addition, it is also possible to diagnose other pathologies such as condyle fractures and fibro-osseous ankylosis of the joint using different viewing planes.

A 3D reconstruction gives a general overview of the TMJ, which is sometimes very helpful in surgical planning in cases of severe morphological abnormalities of the condyle. Examinations of the joint carried out with the mouth open can be really helpful in diagnosing internal derangement of the joint. Here, CBCT has a limited role, as the interarticular disc is not visualized in the image. Second, to know the range and type of movement of the condyle, a second scan of the patient is obtained in an open mouth position. It should always be taken into consideration that a second scan in an open mouth position exposes the patient to additional radiation exposure.

(a)

(b)

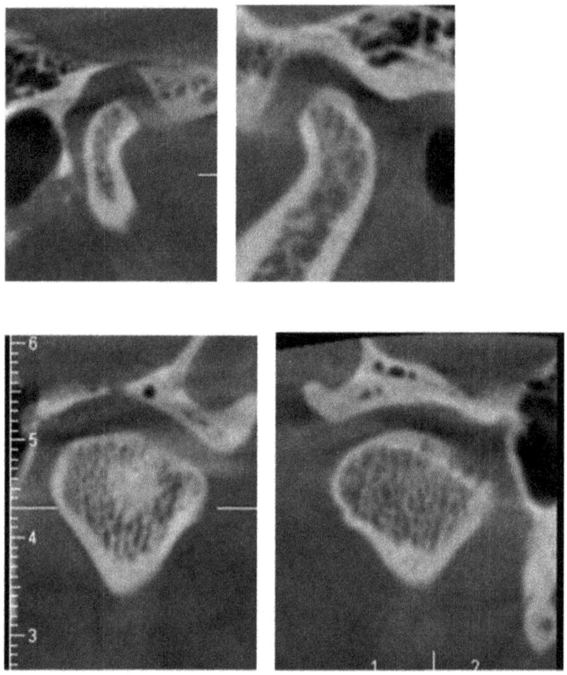

Figure Case 4.2. (a) Sagittal sections showing flattening of the right and left condyles. (b) Coronal sections showing subcortical sclerosis of the right condyle and irregular cortical erosions of the left condyle.

Illustrative case 02*: *Chasing the TMJ

A 40-year-old lady, a doctor by profession, walked in for a CBCT scan as she was troubled with pain in her TM joint. A brief history revealed that there was continuous pain of severe intensity in the both TM joints. The movements of the mandible were not restricted. Chewing food was difficult due to pain. It was seen that the supero-anterior articulating surfaces of the left and right TMJs exhibited mild flattening. Subcortical sclerosis was noted in the right condyle. Irregular cortical erosions of the superior surface of the left condyle were noted. The left and right condyles exhibited adequate anterior translation in the mandibular open mouth position as they were seen to lie below the articular eminence. The radiographic findings were consistent with bone remodeling and early degenerative disease of the right and left condyles (figure case 4.2).

4.5.7 Airway analysis

A physician may evaluate the airway space in a 2D manner using lateral cephalograms. This yields limited information due to the use of a flat projection in the sagittal plane. CBCT can make a 3D projection of the airway available. It is also possible to measure the volume of the airway and the sinuses. This information is particularly relevant in cases of patients with mouth breathing habits and airway obstruction (sleep apnea).

4.5.8 Evaluating impacted teeth

The prevailing technique is to obtain two conventional radiographs perpendicular to each other and then identify the location of the tooth. In addition, the tube-shift technique provides the arbitrary location of the tooth based upon the movement of the objects in consideration. CBCT is precise in determining the labio/buccal and palatal/lingual position of the impacted tooth, the angulation and orientation of the impacted tooth, and its proximity to the roots of the adjacent teeth and anatomic structures, especially the mandibular canal.

The extraction of impacted mandibular third molars may lead to dysesthesia due to damage to the inferior Alveolar nerve. It is known that the risk increases if there is direct contact between the nerve and the tooth root. In CBCT, the nerve marking tool helps to accurately locate the entire course of the inferior alveolar nerve canal through the body of the mandible. It is also beneficial in identifying the presence of accessory nerves. It thus provides a clear picture to the operating surgeon who in turn can take precautions to avoid iatrogenic trauma to the inferior alveolar nerve during surgical extraction of mandibular third molars.

Fracture of the lingual cortical plate and accidental displacement of the third molar and its root fragments are uncommon but serious complications of third molar surgery. Perforation of the lingual cortical plate during third molar surgery can create direct access to the submandibular space. Such complications occur when the tooth is lingually placed or oriented. CBCT is a very valuable tool for identifying the relationship between the impacted third molar and the lingual cortical bone and for evaluating the thickness of the cortex.

Illustrative case 03: Finding wisdom with an impacted wisdom tooth

A 38-year-old male patient was referred for CBCT evaluation as a panoramic radiograph showed a horizontally impacted mandibular third molar superimposed over the inferior alveolar nerve canal with well-defined periapical radiopacity. CBCT revealed that tooth 3–8 had two roots which appeared to be fused together. There was a well-defined radiodense mass associated with the roots of 3–8, which extended from the coronal third of the root and had formed an ovoid-shaped entity in its periapical region. This entity was surrounded by a thin hypodense lining of variable width. The density appeared to be comparable to that of dentin/cementum. The left inferior alveolar nerve canal (IANC) was seen inferior to the horizontally impacted 3–8. Posteriorly, the radiodensity seems to have enveloped and pushed the IANC along its course towards the buccal cortical bone. Obliteration of the root apex was noted. No evidence of root resorption. A radiographic diagnosis of benign cementoblastoma with a differential diagnosis of atypical hypercementosis was given (figure case 4.3).

4.5.9 Dentomaxillofacial pathology

Benign tumors: CBCT is the most useful tool for the identification and diagnosis of various oral and maxillofacial pathologies. Intra- and extraoral radiographs can only cover the entire extent of the pathology in the superoinferior and mesiodistal planes. Observation of the third dimension (buccolingual/palatal plane) is only possible in CBCT. The multiplanar views in CBCT provide vital information

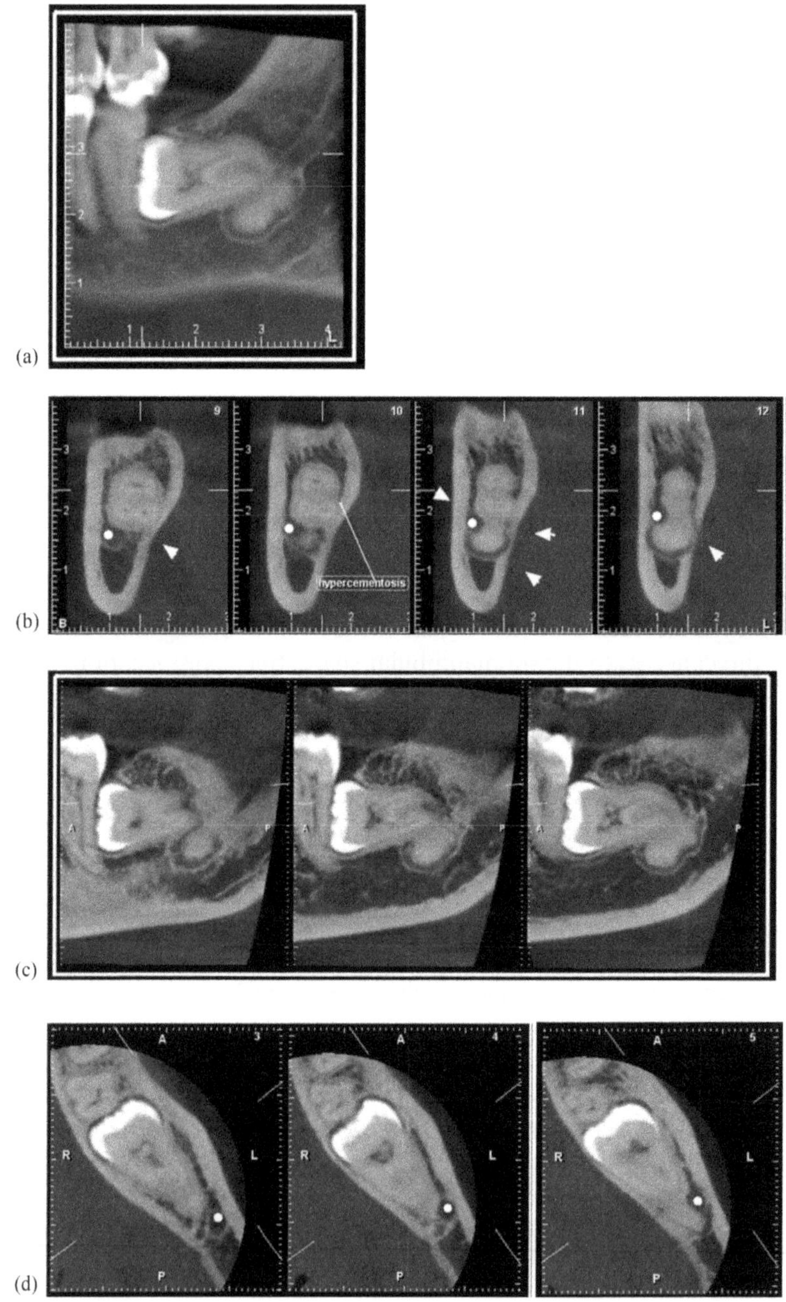

Figure Case 4.3. (a) A cropped panoramic view. (b) Coronal sections at 2 mm intervals showing the hyperdense mass abutting the inferior alveolar nerve canal. (c) Sagittal sections at 2 mm intervals showing mass with a density comparable to that of dentin/cementum and with a thin hypodense lining of variable width surrounding it. (d) Axial sections for the same patient showing the relationship between the inferior alveolar nerve and the horizontally impacted third molar.

about the presence and extent of bone resorption, sclerosis of the adjacent bone, the extent of cortical bone expansion with or without perforation, the extent and type of periosteal bone deposition, and internal or external calcifications (figures 4.20–4.24).

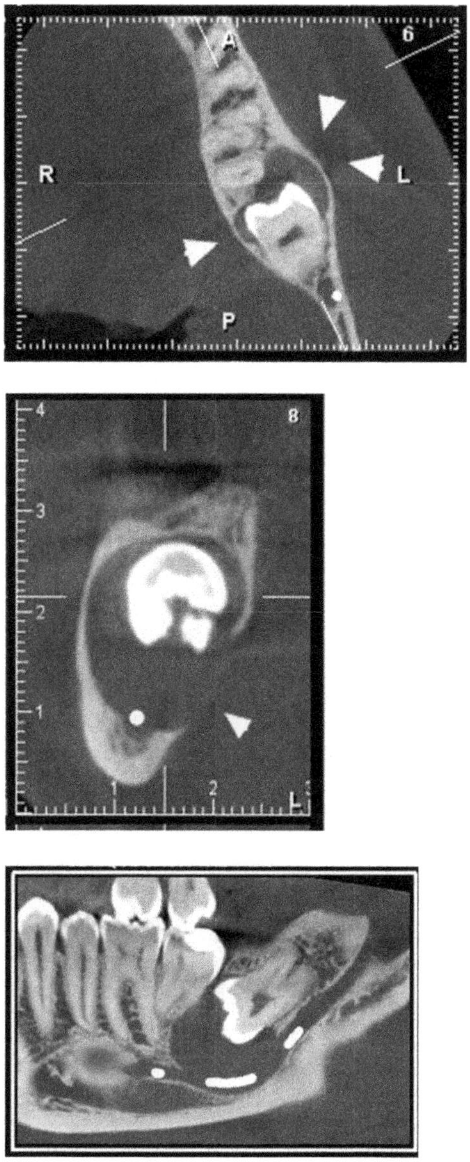

(a)
(b)
(c)

Figure 4.20. (a) A horizontally impacted mandibular third molar with well-defined pericoronal hypodensity, which is most likely to be a dentigerous cyst. The buccal cortical bone expansion is well displayed. (b) Cross sections through the body of the mandible showing an impacted tooth with thinning and perforation of the lingual cortical bone and loss of the roof of the inferior alveolar nerve canal. (c) A sagittal section showing inferior displacement of the inferior alveolar nerve canal with destruction of its roof and distal tipping of the second molar.

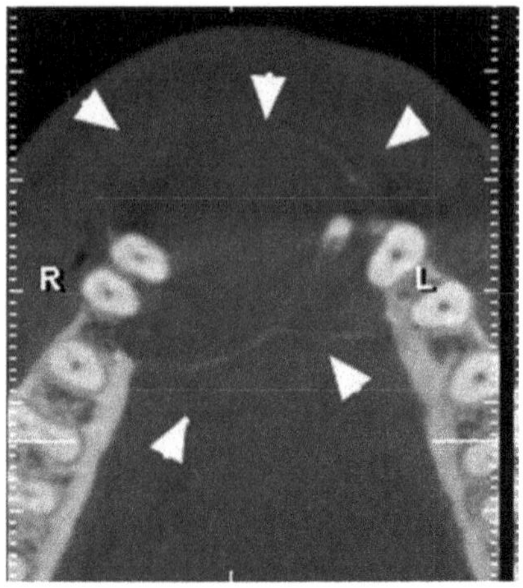

Figure 4.21. A case of anterior mandibular ameloblastoma showing severe expansion of the labial and lingual cortical bone. The massive expansion and osteolysis makes the thin expanded cortex almost invisible on the scan. Areas of perforation noted labially.

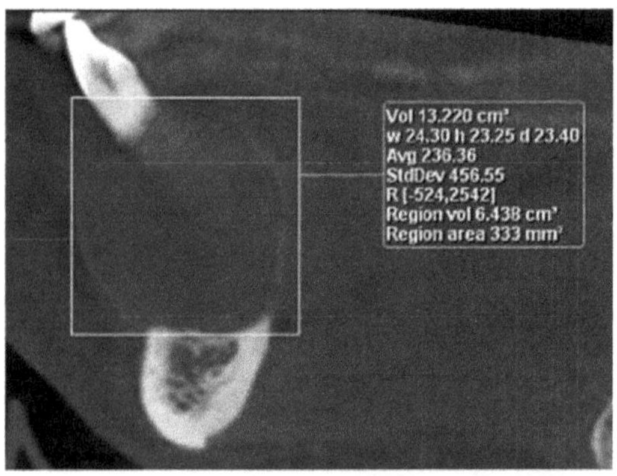

Figure 4.22. A volume and area measurement of the osteolytic entity assessed in CBCT for the same case.

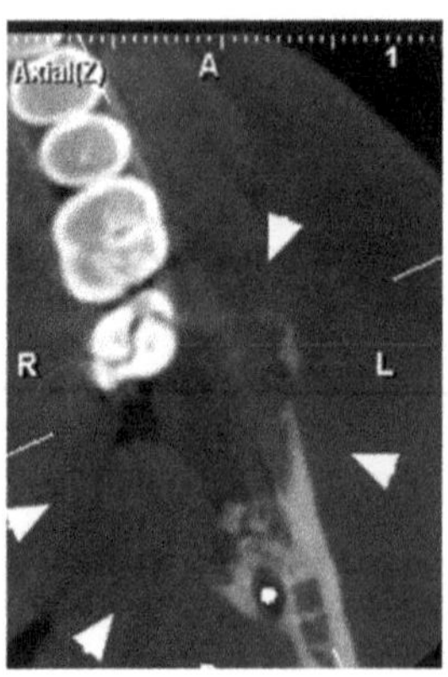

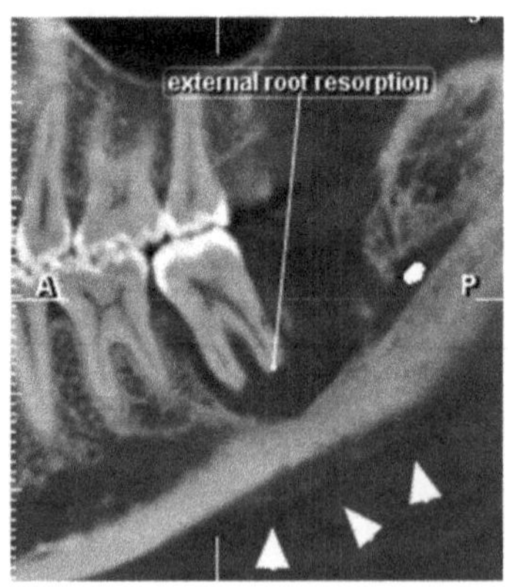

Figure 4.23. A CBCT image of a mandible showing a case of osteosarcoma of the mandible. The axial and sagittal sections show bone destruction with irregular margins; the sagittal section displays a 'tooth floating in air' appearance.

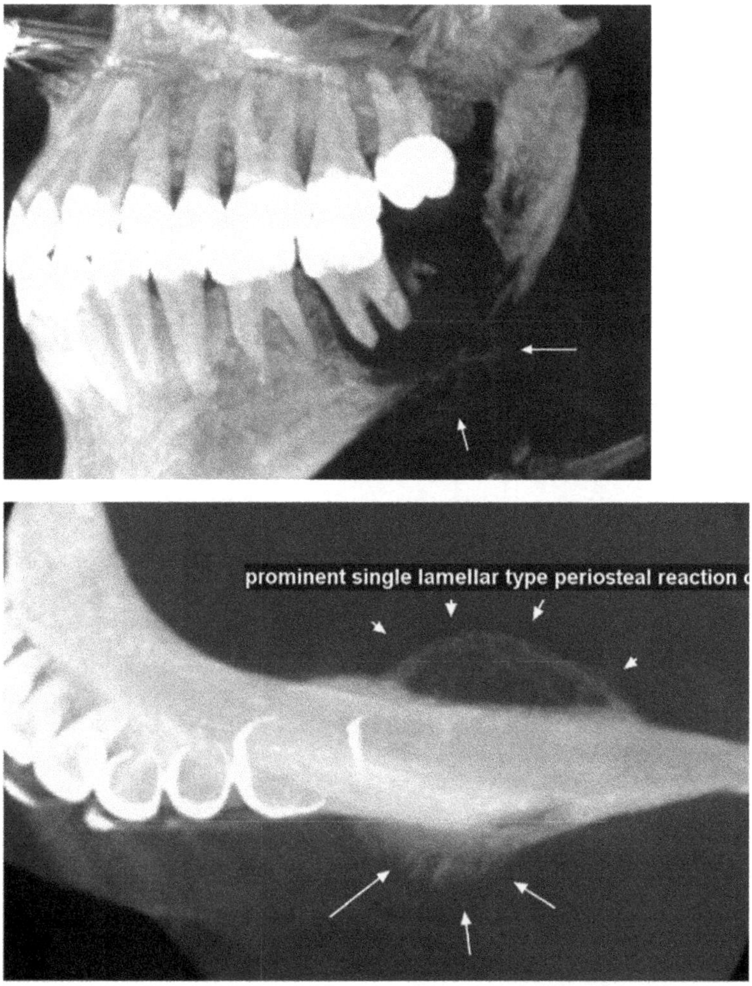

Figure 4.24. A reconstructed 3D view for the same patient showing a single lamellar-type periosteal reaction on the lingual aspect and a spiculated pattern due to periosteal reaction on the buccal aspect.

Illustrative case 04: Mysterious swelling in the hard palate

A 29-year-old male was referred for CBCT of the maxilla. He complained of pain and swelling over the hard palate. The following are the CBCT findings. A well-defined, unilocular, osteolytic entity was noted in the maxilla extending from the periapical regions of teeth 1–6 to 2–3. The margins were well defined, regular, and thinly corticated and appeared to be scalloped. There was marked buccal and minimal palatal cortical bone expansion. Thinning of expanded cortices was noted with areas of perforation on the distal aspect of this entity. Multiple irregular calcifications forming a concentric pattern were noted within this entity below the floor of the nasal cavity. A horizontally impacted 1–3 was noted above the periapical region of 1–4 and 1–5 and was seen to contact the apical root surfaces of 1–4 and 1–5; its root was positioned distally and towards the buccal cortical bone. Loss of the lamina dura was noted in relation to 1–6, 1–5, 1–4, 1–2, 1–1, 2–1, 2–2, and 2–3. There was evidence of external root resorption of 1–6, 1–5, 1–4 and 1–2. The root of 1–4 was displaced in the distal and buccal directions and the root of 1–2 was displaced mesially. The osteolytic lesion had caused thinning and perforation of the nasopalatine nerve canal. Superior displacement and thinning of the floor of the maxillary sinus and nasal cavity floor were observed.

It was agreed that the findings were suggestive of a benign odontogenic tumor, most likely to be an adenomatoid odontogenic tumor with differential diagnosis of ameloblastoma. However, a remote possibility of a collateral variant of dentigerous cyst could not be ruled out, as the epicenter of the lesion was located on the lateral aspect of the impacted canine (figure case 4.4).

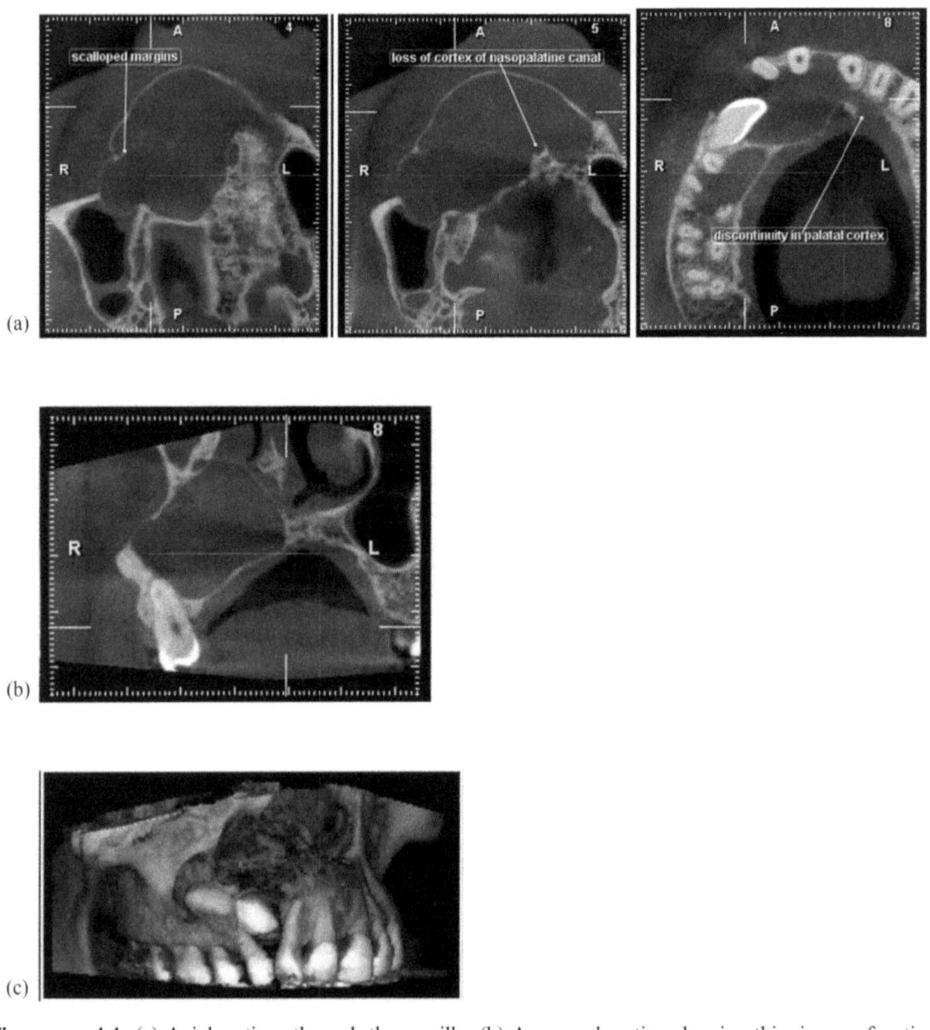

Figure case 4.4. (a) Axial sections through the maxilla. (b) A coronal section showing thinning, perforation, and superior displacement of the nasal cavity floor. (c) A 3D reconstruction of the maxilla showing the position and orientation of the impacted canine.

Illustrative Case 05: Surprised by sclerosis

A well-defined focus of granular bone was noted in the alveolar bone in relation to the apical aspect of the distal root of 3–6 and superior to the IANC. It measured 8.64 mm (anteroposterior) × 7.74 mm (buccolingual) x 9.01 mm (superoinferior). There was no evidence of a radiolucent rim around the periphery. The hyperdensity was surrounded by a thin corticated margin. The margins were regular and well defined. On the lingual aspect, this entity appeared to be continuous with the lingual cortical bone as seen on axial sections. There was no evidence of displacement of the IANC. There was no evidence of cortical bone expansion. The surrounding alveolar trabeculae displayed a normal architecture. The radiographic findings reflect the presence of a focal cemento–osseous dysplasia at site 3–6 (dormant phase). Differential diagnoses include idiopathic osteoscleorosis and cementoblastoma (figure case 4.5).

Osteomyelitis: the features of malignancy and osteomyelitis can look similar in plain radiographs and can cause difficulty in diagnosis. In cases of acute infection, CBCT scans are not useful, as the early infection produces no bony changes that can be appreciated on radiographs or scanned images. In cases of chronic infection, the bone appears to be of mixed density. Periosteal bone deposition resulting from chronic osteomyelitis is readily seen on CBCT. These changes may or may not be seen in traditional occlusal radiographs owing to incorrect exposure factors and angulation. From a surgical perspective, CBCT is able to display even the smallest bony sequestra seen in osteomyelitis which needs surgical debridement.

Mastoiditis and elongated styloid process: chronic or subacute mastoiditis may occur as a result of incomplete treatment of otitis media or middle ear infections. The mastoid process is a part of the temporal bone. It is included in the edge of most volumes of routine CBCT scans. Radiographically, the mastoid process is easy to

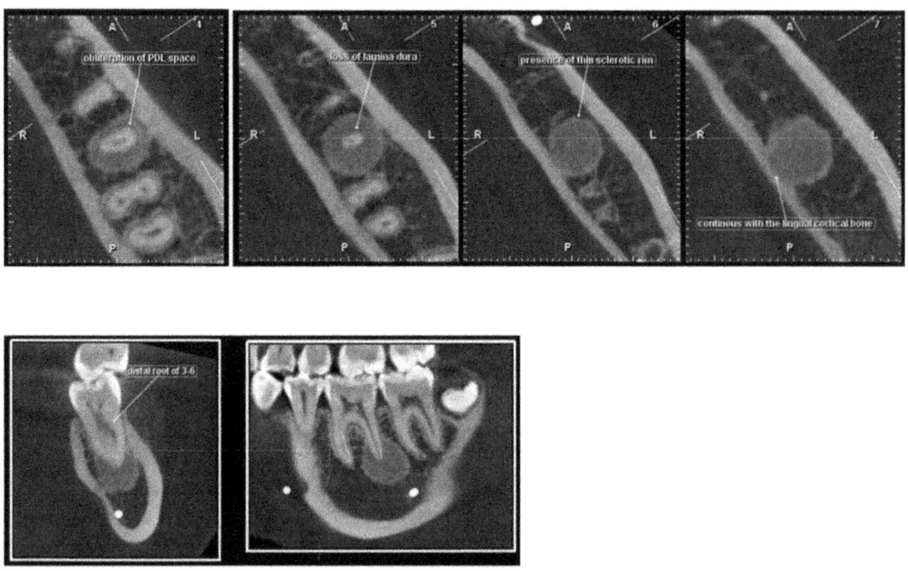

Figure Case 4.5. (a) Axial sections at 2 mm intervals. (b) The coronal and sagittal sections.

spot, as it is made up of intricate trabeculae and interwoven air spaces. Another interesting yet seldom advised application of CBCT is evaluation of the styloid process. The styloid process is very well seen in skull radiographs, but its angulation and orientation are not decipherable. CT is also preferred but at the expense of causing higher radiation exposure to the patient. The CBCT discovery of an elongated styloid process is described in the illustrative case below.

Illustrative case 06*: *Eagle's syndrome.

A 25-year-old woman complained of pain in the neck and throat region and was referred for a CBCT scan. The left styloid process was thin and slender. It was seen to be in two separate parts; (1) the tympanohyal styolohyal part of the process, which was attached to the base of the skull and measured 8.19 mm and (2) the styolohyal part of the process which measured 14.25 mm. The right styloid process is comparatively slightly thick. It is seen in two separate parts; (1) the tympanohyal styolohyal part of the process which is attached to the base of the skull near the and measures 7.15 mm and (2) the styolohyal part of the process which measured 16.24 mm. This was a case of a bilateral elongated and segmented styloid process (figure case 4.6).

Maxillary sinus: for a dentist, identifying the condition of the maxillary sinuses is of the utmost importance for implant planning, endodontic procedures, and to rule out sinus pathology as a cause of orofacial pain. ENT specialists can also obtain valuable information from paranasal sinus CBCT scans. Sinusitis is a very common mucosal inflammatory disease affecting the maxillary sinus which can be detected by identifying an increase in the thickness of the soft-tissue shadow within the maxillary sinus. CBCT images are also very helpful in identifying mucous retention cysts, antral polyps, sinonasal polyps, oro-antral fistula, and malignancy of the maxillary sinus. CBCT images are dependable for determinations of the size and margin of the mass, the status of the sinus wall, and blockage of the ostium. A major limitation is the poor contrast of the displayed soft-tissue density. Sinus masses may be composed of different types of soft tissue with or without fluid accumulation. The sinus fluid may be a thin watery secretion, blood, or purulent material. In CBCT images, a shadow of mass in the sinus has uniform density. Therefore, the differentiation of this density as either fluid or a soft-tissue mass is not possible (figure 4.25).

Illustrative Case 07: A foreign body in the maxillary sinus

A 32-year-old lady was referred for a CBCT scan. She complained of pain over the maxillary sinus region. CBCT revealed that the walls of the left maxillary sinus appeared intact, except that there was a continuity breach in the floor of the sinus. The was evidence of oro-antral communication covered by a soft-tissue density shadow measuring 1.21 mm at the level of the alveolar ridge in the 2–6 region. There was moderate thickening of the sinus mucosa in relation to the floor of the sinus.

Evidence was noted of three separate highly attenuating radiodense foreign bodies (2700–3300 HU) which appeared to be embedded in the mucosal thickening in the floor of the left maxillary sinus; these measured approximately 3.95 mm, 2.75 mm, and 2.45 mm in their directions of greatest length. An enlarged ostium was noted within the

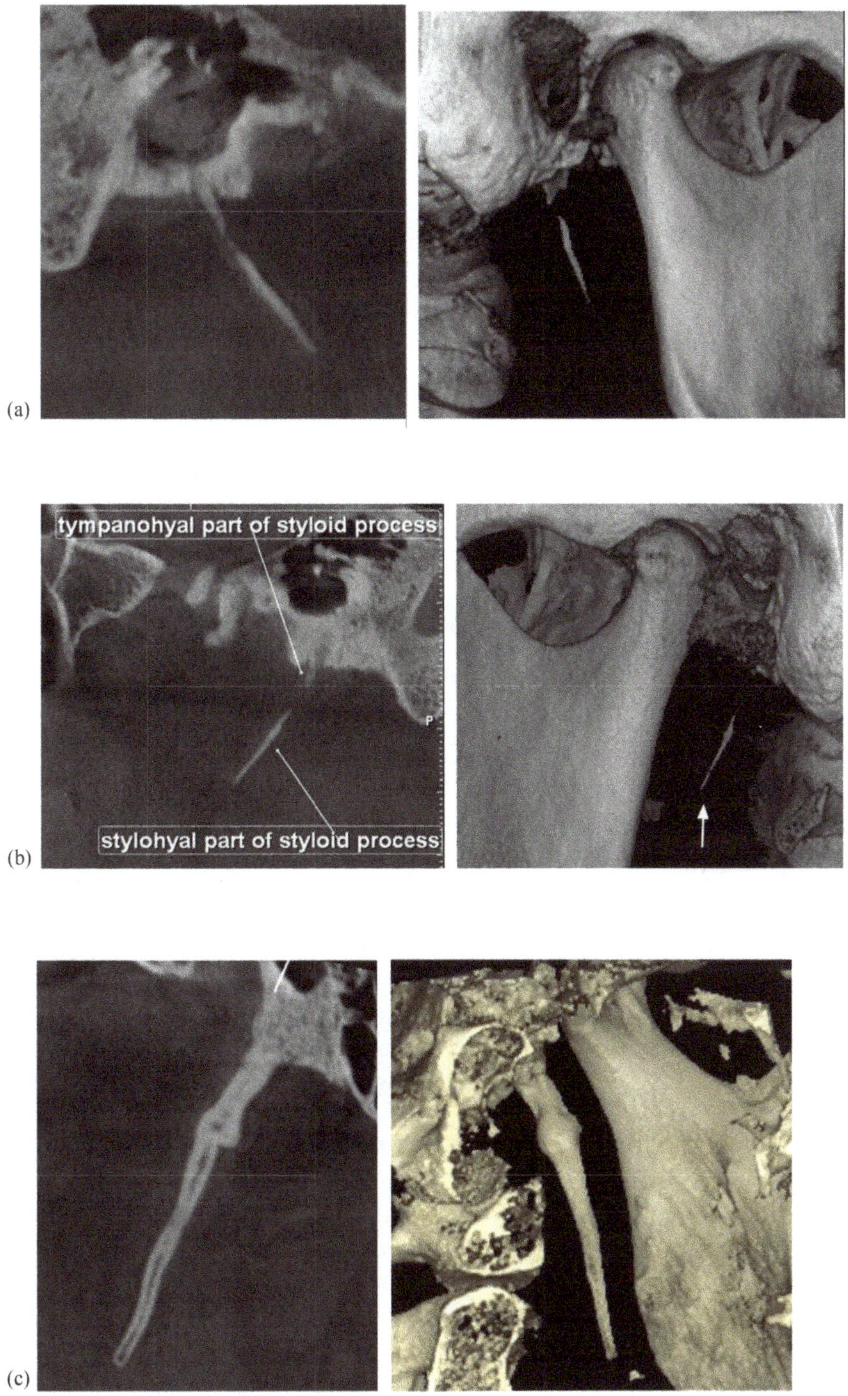

Figure case 4.6. (a) A sagittal section of the right styloid process along with a 3D reconstruction. (b) A sagittal section of the left styloid process along with a 3D reconstruction. (c) In another patient, the styloid process was intact and elongated.

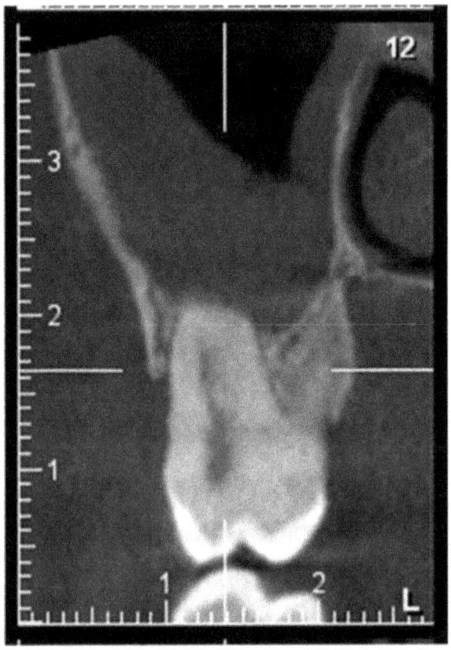

Figure 4.25. Thick soft-tissue density seen in the floor of the maxillary sinus; it is suggestive of chronic maxillary sinusitis.

medial wall of the left maxillary sinus. Osseous calcifications were noted along the posterior lateral wall (figure case 4.7).

Cleft palate: Treatment planning for cleft lip and palate patients entails unique considerations. Due to their young ages and the high radiation exposure involved, a CT scan is always not favorable. For such patients it is important to obtain detailed imaging of the osseous cleft, teeth, and unerupted tooth germs for orthodontic and surgical planning. CBCT allows better evaluation of the dental age, arch segment positioning, and estimation of cleft sizes. The following case is a cleft palate case showing CBCT imaging and surgical planning.

Illustrative case 08: A young lady with a beautiful smile

A 22-year-old woman was referred for CBCT of the maxilla to evaluate a cleft palate. The results showed the presence of a unilateral cleft in the alveolar bone on the right side of maxilla starting at the 1–2 region and progressing posteriorly towards the end of the hard palate. This cleft had caused loss of the floor of the nasal cavity on the right side, causing oro-nasal communication. It had also caused loss of the lateral wall of the incisive canal (figure case 4.8).

Salivary glands: Visualizing the ductal system of the major salivary glands has always been a challenge for clinicians. Sialography is a procedure in which a contrast medium is injected into the major salivary glands via the primary duct and

(a)
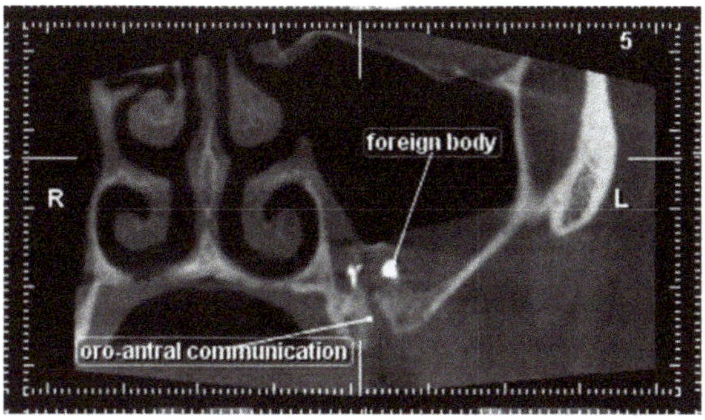

(b)
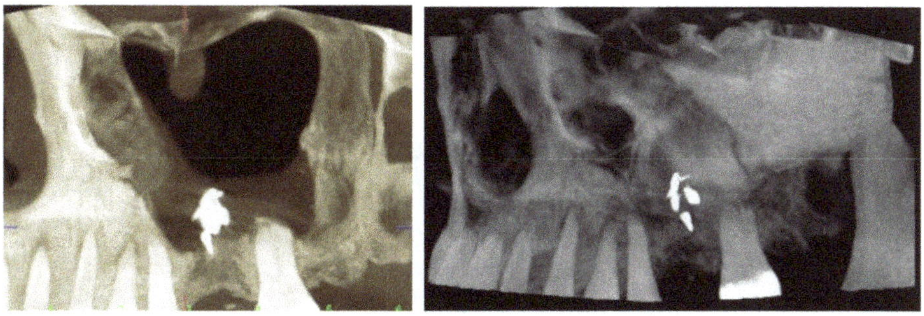

(c)
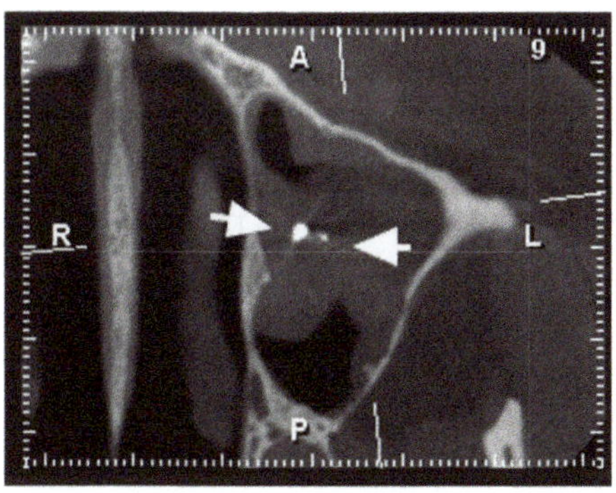

Figure Case 4.7. (a) A coronal section through the nasal cavity and the maxillary sinus showing an enlarged ostium, foreign bodies, and sinusitis. (b) A 3D reconstruction. (c) An axial section through the maxillar sinus helped to localize the position of the foreign body.

radiographic images are obtained. Sialography can also have a therapeutic effect by dislodging small sialoliths and mucous plugs from the ducts. Indications of sialography are sialoliths, sialadenitis, and space-occupying lesions in the major salivary glands. CBCT sialography definitely provides the clinician with more information than conventional 2D sialography; its major advantage is the ability to view the gland and the ductal system in different planes and angles. CBCT helps

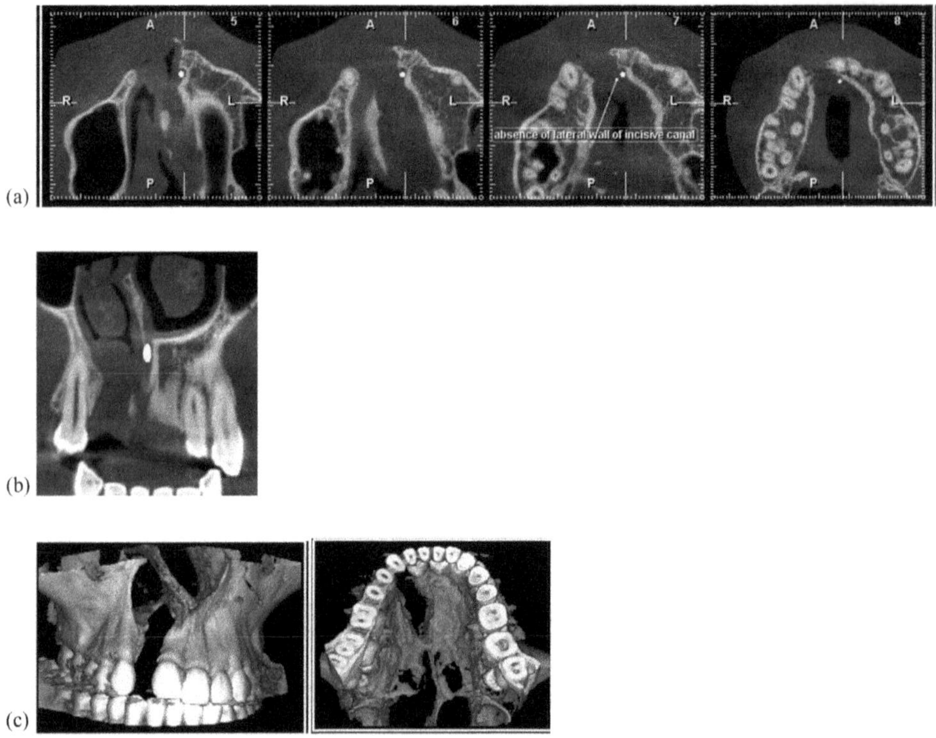

Figure Case 4.8. (a) Axial sections at 2 mm intervals. (b) A coronal section showing the cleft, the absence of a nasal cavity floor on right side, and partial absence of the cortex of the incisive nerve canal. (c) Reconstructed 3D views for the same patient.

to visualize the ducts with great detail, which is otherwise unavailable in conventional 2D sialography. Due to the high resolution of CBCT, it is possible to identify the tertiary and fourth-order ducts as well. It is also possible to carry out volumetric analysis. The contrast dye produces heavy streaking or beam hardening artifacts (see section 4.6), which makes it difficult to read the details. However, this can be overcome by using the artifact reduction or correction tools integrated into the software.

Illustrative case 09: Exploring the undiscovered

The following are CBCT sialography findings for two different patients. Patient X had a history of extraoral preauricular swelling for three years and intraoral pus discharge from the Stenson's duct. After the inflammatory changes subsided post-antibiotic therapy, CBCT sialography of the parotid gland was performed. This revealed the presence of an accessory parotid gland, the sausage string appearance of the primary duct (sialodochitis), and globular sialectesia of the acini (figure case 4.9).

Patient Y was a known case of Sjögren's syndrome who had marked xerostomia in the oral cavity. CBCT revealed narrowing of the primary duct and destruction of the tertiary duct and the acini of the parotid gland.

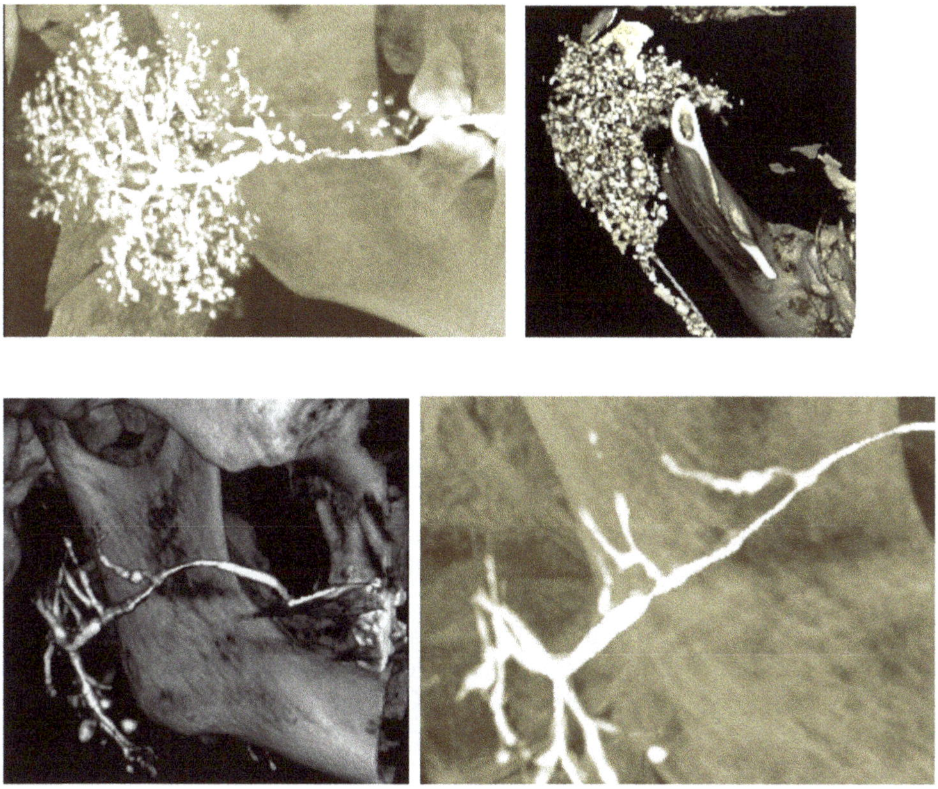

(a)

(b)

Figure Case 4.9. (a) The sausage string appearance of the primary duct (sialodochitis) and globular sialectesia of the acini. (b) Narrowing of the primary duct and destruction of the tertiary duct and the acini.

4.6 CBCT artifacts

It is now well established that CBCT has been accepted as a useful tool for diagnosis and treatment planning in dentistry. The other side of the coin is that CBCT imaging has some drawbacks, such as artifacts. Artifacts are discrepancies between the reconstructed visual image and the actual content of the subject; they degrade the quality of CBCT images, making them diagnostically unusable. In addition, structures that do not exist in the subject may appear within the images. Such artifacts are produced because of various factors such as patient motion and the image capture and reconstruction processes. To optimize image quality, every user should be aware of their presence; it is also necessary to understand the types of artifacts, how they are caused, and methods that can reduce or eliminate them. This section aims to discuss and review the existing knowledge about the artifacts associated with CBCT images.

There are three types of artifacts:

(a) Physics-based artifacts
(b) Scanner-based artifacts
(c) Patient-related artifacts

4.6.1 Physics-based artifacts

The primary cone beam is polychromatic in nature, which means it is made up of x-ray photons of various wavelengths and energies. As this polychromatic beam passes through the patient's tissue, the low-energy x-ray photons are attenuated in the tissue. Thus, a greater percentage of high-energy x-ray photons hits the detector. The software uses the Feldkamp algorithm to process the data obtained by the detector. However, this algorithm assumes that the primary beam is monochromatic. This leads to the assignment of incorrect gray scale values for areas within the subject. The presence of extremely high-density objects in the FOV, for example metal restorations or dental implants, leads to excessive beam attenuation. The resultant images have dark areas and white streaks, which are known as beam hardening artifacts. There are two types of beam hardening artifacts, namely cupping artifacts and streaking artifacts [11]. The following measures can be adopted to reduce the beam hardening artifacts (figure 4.26).

- Reducing the FOV: excluding metal objects from the scan by choosing a limited FOV eliminates beam hardening artifacts.
- Collimation and modification of patient positioning (separation of dental arches).
- Added filtration: a flat piece of metal is used to 'preharden' the beam by filtering out the lower-energy photons before the beam passes through the patient.
- Beam hardening correction software: CBCT artifact reduction algorithms are introduced within the reconstruction process. However, these algorithms are computationally demanding and require increased reconstruction times. Metal artifact reduction software is sometimes limited because, although streaking is removed when it is far from metal implants, loss of detail still remains around the metal–tissue interface, which is often the main area of diagnostic interest.

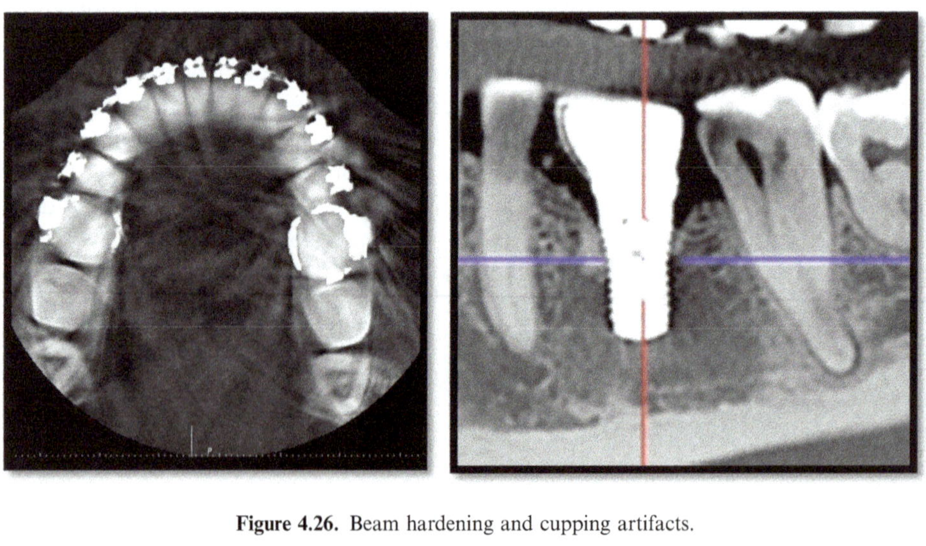

Figure 4.26. Beam hardening and cupping artifacts.

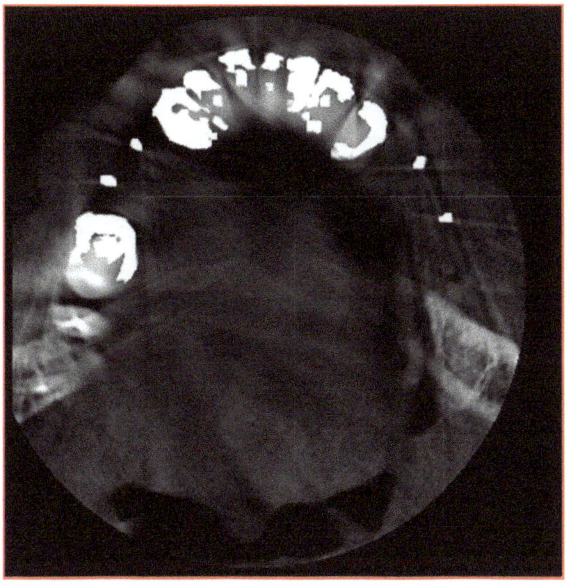

Figure 4.27. The photon starvation effect.

Photon starvation artifacts constitute another type of physics-based artifact. They occur when insufficient photons reach the detector. This can cause streaking in the resulting images due to the presence of high-attenuation areas. Such images have high noise. These artifacts can be reduced by milliamperage modulation. In this method, the tube current is automatically varied during the course of each rotation; this allows sufficient photons to pass through the widest parts of the patient without administering an unnecessary dose to the narrower parts. Adaptive filtration also helps to reduce the streaking in photon-starved images (figure 4.27). This software correction method smooths the attenuation profile in areas of high attenuation before the image is reconstructed [11].

Aliasing artifacts are physics-based artifacts caused by the undersampling of structures within the subject by the cone beam unit's detector. Aliasing artifacts appear as slightly wavy lines that diverge outwards towards the periphery of a cone beam image and form a 'moiré pattern. (Figure 4.28)' Aliasing artifacts can be minimized by acquiring the largest possible number of projections per rotation. For some scanners, this can only be achieved by using a slower rotation speed, while for others, the number of projections is independent of the rotational speed (figure 4.28). Aliasing can be reduced using specialized high-resolution techniques, such as a quarter-detector shift or a flying focal spot, which manufacturers employ to increase the number of samples within a projection [12].

4.6.2 Scanner-based artifacts

Ring artifacts are generated when the detector element is defective or misaligned with the x-ray source. This generates a faulty attenuation value as it travels the arc

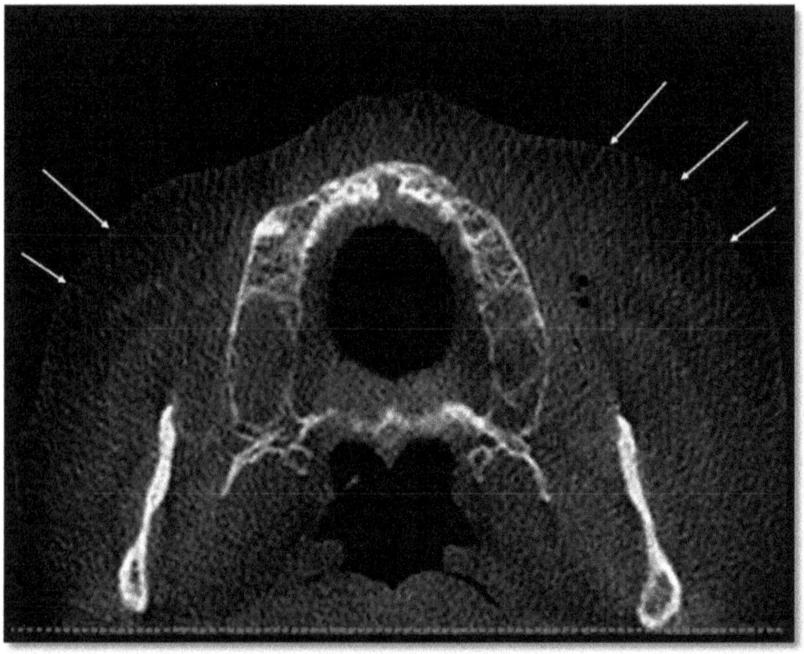

Figure 4.28. A moiré pattern.

around the subject, thereby producing a ring-like artifact (Figure 4.29). These artifacts are commonly seen in axial projections and are centered about the rotational axis of the imaging system. The presence of circular artifacts in an image is an indication that the detector needs recalibration or may need repair services [11]. Selecting the correct scan field of view may reduce the artifact by using calibration data that fit more closely to the patient anatomy. All modern scanners use solid-state detectors, but their potential to produce ring artifacts is reduced by software that characterizes and corrects detector variations (figure 4.29).

4.6.3 Patient-related artifacts

In CBCT, the patient's jaw movement or swallowing movements affect the sharpness of the entire volume data. Motion artifacts are common because of the relatively long acquisition times. They appear as double outlines of corticated surfaces in the reconstructed image. One way to minimize motion artifacts is to reduce the scan time by decreasing the number of basis images used to reconstruct the 3D volume, which reduces overall image quality. However, if the resulting image is compatible with many diagnostic tasks, then it is a good option for patients who make involuntary movements [12]. Essentially, paddles are positioned against the patient's temples or an open face plate is provided on which the patient rests his or her forehead to reduce head movements. Having the patient sit in a chair and lowering the unit to the patient will also help to reduce the chance of patient motion.

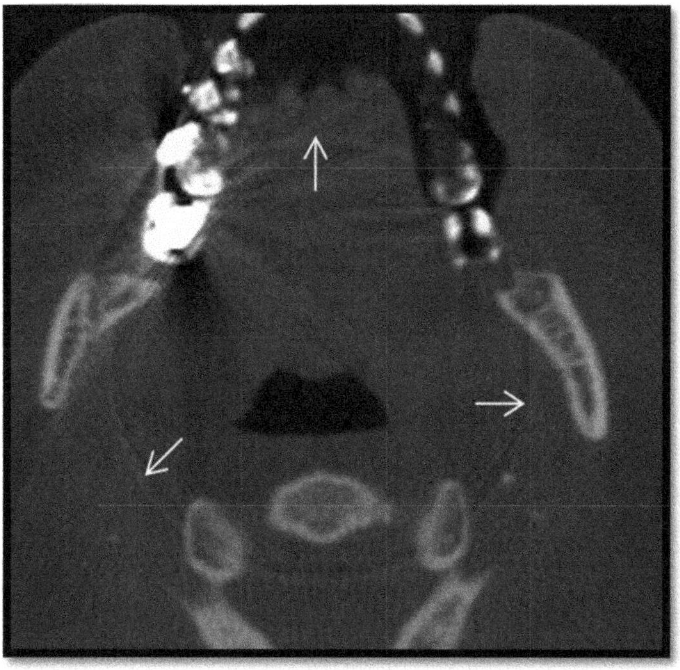

Figure 4.29. A ring artifact.

4.7 Conclusions

CBCT, a relatively advanced imaging modality, has been widely used in dentomaxillofacial diagnosis over the last decade because of its multiple advantages over 2D and other 3D imaging modalities. It produces submillimetre resolution images with minimal to no magnification, thereby improving diagnostic accuracy. The effective radiation doses for CBCT are typically far less than the levels required for clinical spiral CT due to the ability to choose the size of FOV and the reduction in scan time. Although it is easily accessible and a cost-effective option, CBCT imaging should be used judiciously and only as an adjuvant tool to the patient history and clinical examination.

Acknowledgments

The cases and the CBCT images included in the chapter were provided courtesy of the Department of Oral Medicine and Radiology, Goa Dental College and Hospital, Bambolim, Goa and Raghuwanshi's Digital Diagnostic Centre, St. Inez, Panjim, Goa.

References and further reading

[1] Baba R *et al* 2002 Comparison of flat-panel detector and image-intensifier detector for cone-beam CT *Comput. Med. Imaging Graph.* **26** 153–8

[2] Mah J and Hatcher D 2003 Current status and future needs in craniofacial imaging *Orthod. Craniofac. Res* **6** 10–6 discussion 179–82

[3] Abramovitch K 2014 Basic Principles of cone beam computed tomography *Dent. Clin. N. Am.* **58** 463–84

[4] Mah J K *et al* 2003 Radiation absorbed in maxillofacial imaging with a new dental Computed tomography device *Oral Surg. Oral Med. Oral Pathol. Oral Radiol. Endod* **96** 508–13

[5] Jacobs R 2011 Dental cone beam CT and its justified use in oral health care *JBR-BTR* **94** 254–65

[6] Miles D A and Danforth R A 2008 A clinician's guide to understanding cone beam volumetric imaging (CBVI). Santa Monica, CA: Academy of Dental Therapeutics and Stomatology

[7] Lofthag-Hansen S, Huumonen S and Gröndahl K *et al* 2007 Limited cone-beam CT and intraoral radiography for the diagnosis of periapical pathology *Oral Surg. Oral Med. Oral Pathol. Oral Radiol. Endod.* **103** 114–19 Epub 2006 Apr 24

[8] Vertucci F J 1984 Root canal anatomy of the human permanent teeth *Oral Surg. Oral Med. Oral Pathol.* **58** 589–99

[9] Terakado M, Hashimoto K and Arai Y *et al* 2000 Diagnostic imaging with newly developed ortho cubic super-high resolution computed tomography (ortho-CT) *Oral Surg. Oral Med. Oral Pathol. Oral Radiol. Endod.* **89** 509–18

[10] Quereshy F A, Savell T A and Palom J M 2008 Applications of cone beam tomography in the practice of oral and maxillofacial surgery *J. Oral Maxillofac. Surg* **66** 791–6

[11] Schulze R, Hail U, Grob D, Bruellmann D D, Dranischnikow E, Schwanecke U and Schoemer E 2011 Artefacts in CBCT: a review *Dentomaxillofac. Radiol.* **40** 265–73

[12] Scott R 2014 Makins; artifacts interfering with interpretation of cone beam computed tomography images *Dent. Clin. N. Am.* **58** 485–95

[13] Scarfe W C and Farman A G 2008 What is cone beam CT and how does it work? *Dent. Clin. N. Am* **52** 707–30

Chapter 5

The application of MRI in dentomaxillofacial pathologies

Manisha M Khorate and Prachi M Desai

Magnetic resonance imaging (MRI) is a noninvasive, three-dimensional modality which uses nonionizing radiation. It thereby avoids the risk of biological damage caused by other 3D imaging techniques which use ionizing radiation.

The principle of MRI is based on presence of a strong and static magnetic field and radio-frequency (RF) pulses and their interaction with protons, particularly the hydrogen atoms present in the human body. Hence, tissues with higher water contents can be visualized with superior contrast in all three imaging planes.

The applications of MRI in dentistry include salivary gland imaging, assessment of the temporomandibular joint (TMJ) articular disc and joint space, the evaluation of soft-tissue masses in the head and neck regions, etc. However, its relatively long scanning time, the claustrophobia of patients, or the presence of biomedical devices such as pacemakers or fixed metal prostheses may present limitations for MRI imaging. This chapter highlights the applications of MRI imaging in dentistry along with its merits and demerits.

5.1 Introduction

- MRI is a noninvasive, three-dimensional imaging modality. It is utilized primarily to evaluate pathologies involving the soft tissues, to differentiate between internal structures of varying densities, and to study tissues in their functional state.
- The principle of MRI is based on the presence of a strong and static magnetic field and RF pulses and their interaction with protons, particularly the hydrogen atoms present in the human body. Hence, tissues with higher water contents can be visualized with superior contrast in all three imaging planes [1, 2].

doi:10.1088/978-0-7503-5316-8ch5

- The system uses nonionizing RF electromagnetic radiation in the presence of controlled magnetic fields to obtain high-quality cross-sectional images of the body [3]. It thereby avoids the risk of biological damage caused by other imaging techniques which use ionizing radiation.

5.2 History [3–6]

- 1857–1952—Sir Joseph Larmor described the Larmor relationship.
- 1882—Nicola Tesla discovered the rotating magnetic field for the first time in Budapest.
- 1937—Isidor Isaac Rabi described the phenomenon of NMR for the first time (i.e. the phenomenon of the emission of radio waves by atomic nuclei when exposed to a strong magnetic field).
- 1946—Felix Bloch and Edward Purcell discovered the magnetic resonance phenomenon independently. They were awarded the Nobel Prize in 1952.
- 1973—Paul Lauterbur produced the first magnetic resonance image.
- 1977—Peter Mansfield made the first human scan using an MRI prototype.
- 1977—Raymand Damadian completed the first magnetic resonance (MR) scanner.
- 1980—Bottomley produced the first localized MR image of the heart and brain and thus MRI was developed for clinical use.
- 1987—Dumoulin discovered MR angiography.
- 1990—The primary form of functional MRI was discovered by Seiji Ogawa.
- 1991—Richard Robert Ernst was awarded the Nobel Prize in Chemistry for contributions to the development of the method of high-resolution NMR spectroscopy.
- 2003—Paul C Lauterbur and Sir Peter Mansfield were jointly awarded the Nobel Prize in Physiology or Medicine.

5.3 The basic physics and principle of MRI [7, 8]

The theory of MRI is based on the magnetic properties of the atom. All atomic nuclei consist of protons and neutrons (nucleons), each of which possesses a spin or angular momentum. Nuclei that have evenly paired protons and neutrons produce a net spin of zero, as the spin of each nucleon cancels that of another. Certain atomic nuclei that contain an unpaired proton or neutron, such as the hydrogen nucleus, 1H, or the phosphorus nucleus, 31P, possess a property known as 'spin' (figure 5.1).

In nuclei with unpaired nucleons, a magnetic field is generated due to the electrical charge associated with the spin. This results in each nucleus acting as a magnetic dipole (with north and south poles). In the absence of an external magnetic field, the hydrogen atoms in a sample containing multiple hydrogen atoms are randomly oriented, with the result that the total magnetization of the sample is zero (figure 5.2).

When a strong, external magnetic field (B_0) is applied, the nuclei in the sample align themselves either in parallel with (spin-up) or anti-parallel (spin-down) to the external magnetic field (figure 5.3). The combined effect of these two energy states is

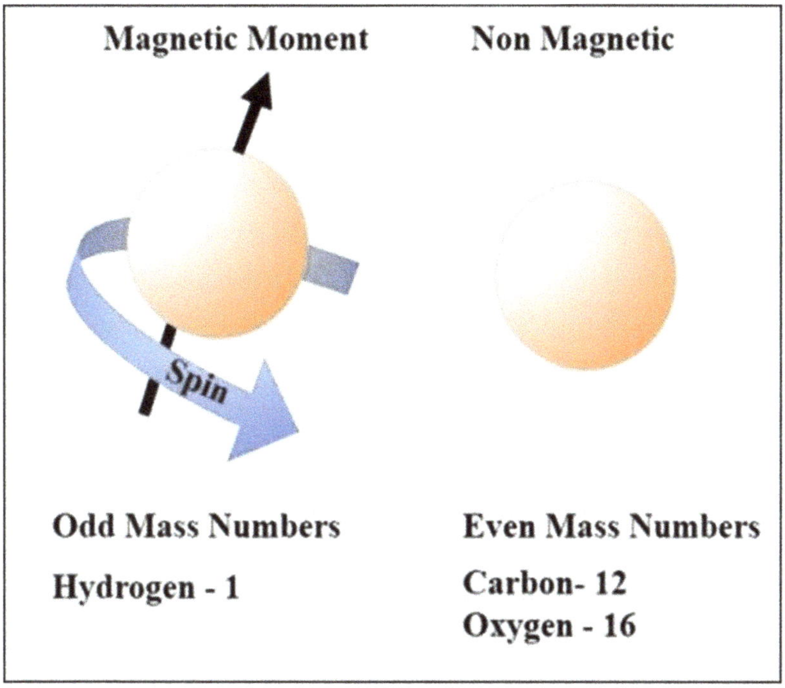

Figure 5.1. The magnetic properties of nuclei.

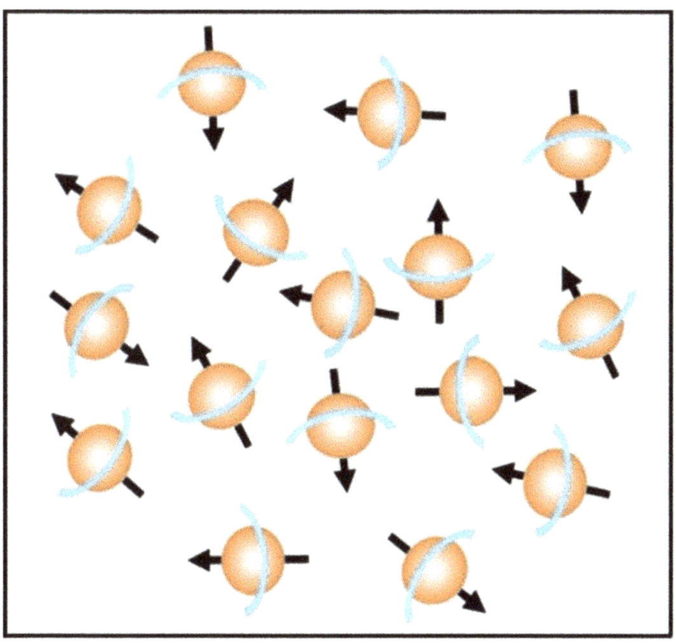

Figure 5.2. The orientation of hydrogen atoms in the absence of an external magnetic field.

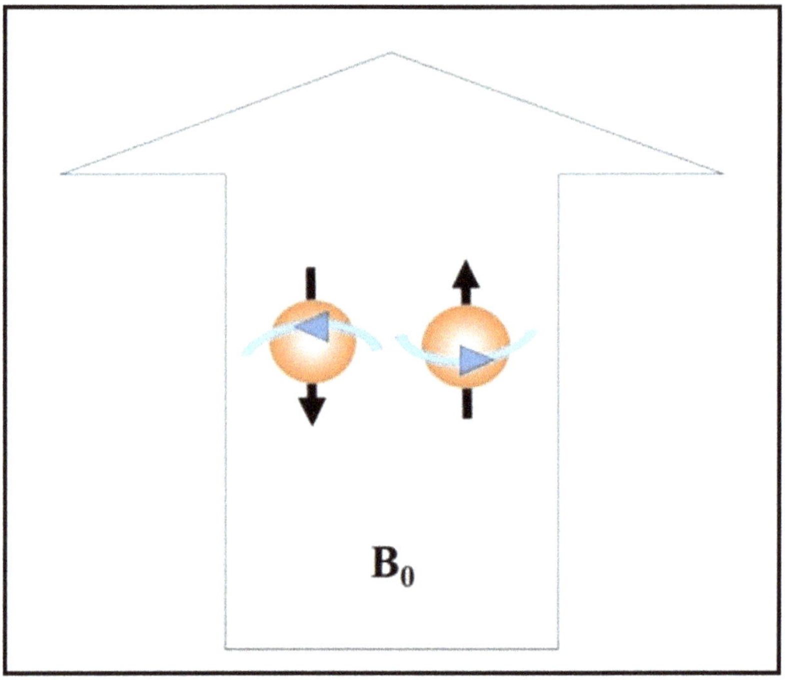

Figure 5.3. Nuclei align in parallel with or anti-parallel to the applied external magnetic field (B_0).

a weak net magnetic moment, or magnetization vector (Mv), which lies parallel to the applied magnetic field [9].

The hydrogen nuclei which *parallel* the external field are considered to be in a lower energy state compared to those which align *anti-parallel*, as more energy is needed to align against the external field direction. Usually, more nuclei prefer to be in the lower energy state and are in the spin-up position.

When B_0 is applied, the north and south poles of the nuclei do not exactly align with the external magnetic field. The axes of spinning protons oscillate or wobble with a slight tilt from a position parallel to the flux of the external magnet. This tilting or wobbling is called precession. The precessing motion is a physical phenomenon that results from an interaction between the magnetic field and the spinning momentum of the nucleus. Precession is often observed in a child's spinning top. A spinning top does not stand vertical for long, but begins to tilt/wobble, or precess. In this case of a spinning top, the precession is caused by an interaction between the Earth's gravitational field and the spinning momentum of the top (figure 5.4) [7].

5.3.1 The Larmor frequency

The velocity of rotation around the field direction is the Larmor frequency. It is specific to the nuclear species and depends on the strength of the external magnetic field. The Larmor frequency of hydrogen is 42.58 MHz in a magnetic field of 1 tesla (T).

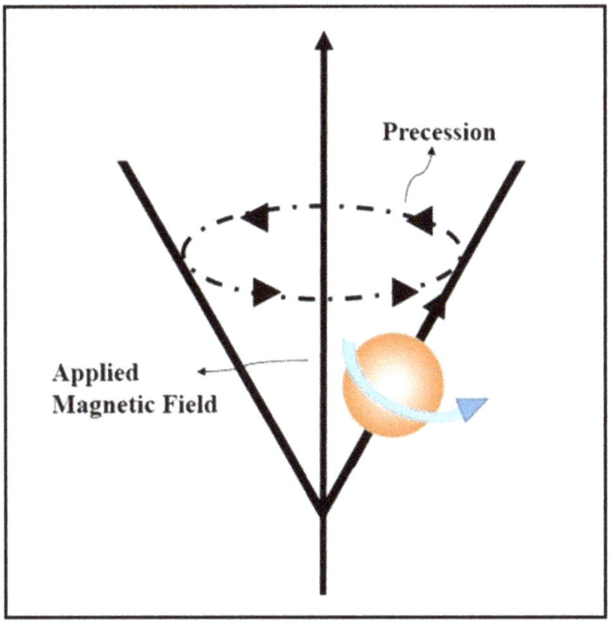

Figure 5.4. Precession: the tilting of the nuclei around the direction of B_0.

One tesla is 10 000 times the strength of the Earth's magnetic field. The magnetic field strengths used for MRI range from 0.1 to 4.0 T [9].

Once a sample of tissue has been placed within the static magnetic field, B_0, a second RF magnetic field B_1 is applied perpendicular to B_0. This results in the excitation of the nuclei that possess spin within B_0. The protons in the tissue that possess a Larmor frequency matching that of B_1 absorb energy and shift or rotate away from the direction induced by B_0. The angle of rotation depends on the duration of the applied RF pulse. If the RF pulse is applied for a sufficient duration, it rotates the net tissue magnetization vector into the XY (i.e. transverse) plane, which is perpendicular to the z-axis (i.e. the longitudinal axis). This causes all protons to precess in phase. This is termed a 'flip angle of 90 degrees' or a '90-degree RF pulse' [9]. The RF energy is usually applied in short pulses, each lasting microseconds. During MRI sequencing, multiple RF pulses of varying intensities can be applied (figures 5.5 and 5.6).

5.3.2 The magnetic resonance signal [10]

The net magnetization of the tissue in the transverse plane and the amount of transverse magnetization that exists at the termination of the RF pulse are equal to the amount of longitudinal magnetization that existed before the pulse. Both are directly proportional to the strength of the static magnetic field and the overall concentration of hydrogen nuclei (proton density) in the tissue. The signal strength also depends on the degree to which hydrogen is bound within a molecule.

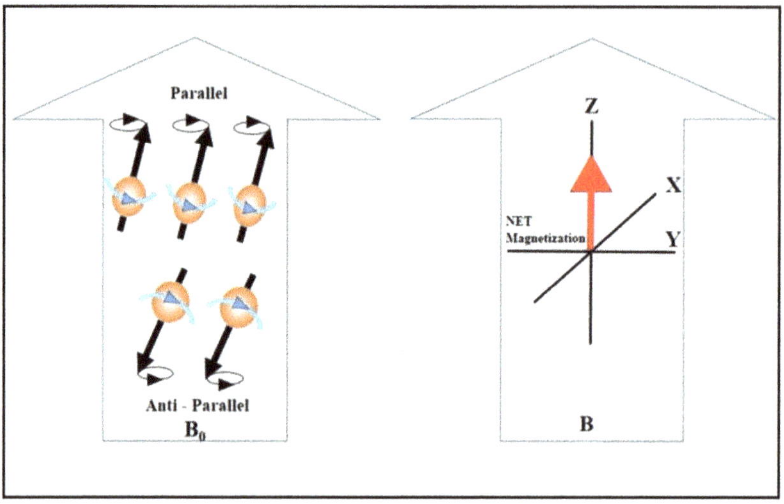

Figure 5.5. NMv.

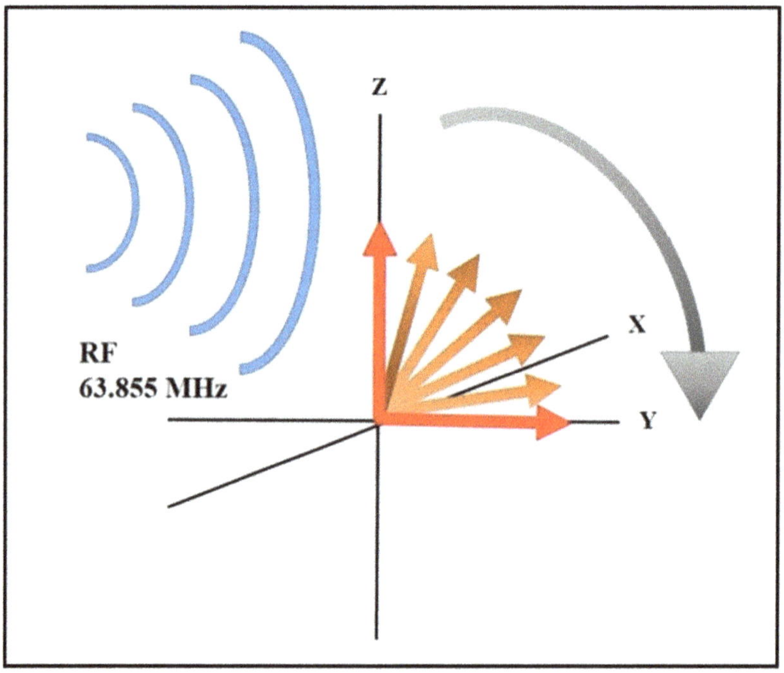

Figure 5.6. A flip angle of 90°.

Tightly bound hydrogen atoms, such as in hydroxyapatite in bone, do not align themselves with the external magnetic field and produce a weak signal. Loosely bound and mobile hydrogen atoms, such as those in soft tissues and liquids, react to the RF pulse and produce a detectable signal at the end of the RF pulse. The concentration of loosely bound hydrogen nuclei available to create the signal is referred to as the proton density or spin density of the tissue in question. The higher the concentration of loosely bound hydrogen atoms, the stronger the transverse magnetization, the stronger the MR signal, and the brighter the corresponding part of the MR image.

When the RF pulse is turned off, the nuclei begin to return to their original lower-energy spin state, a process called relaxation. As some of the high-energy nuclei return to the low-energy state, the longitudinal magnetization, M_Z, returns to its original equilibrium state. In addition, the individual magnetic moments of the protons independently begin to interact with each other and dephase. This dephasing results in a reduction of the magnetization in the transverse plane, M_{XY}, a condition called decay. The loss of transverse magnetization and the dephasing of the hydrogen nuclei causes a loss of intensity of the MR signal. The decreasing voltage recorded in the receiving coil is called the free induction decay (FID) signal.

5.3.3 T1 and T2 relaxation [9, 10]

The relaxation that occurs at the end of the RF pulse results in the recovery of the longitudinal magnetization; this is accomplished by a transfer of energy (spin) from individual hydrogen nuclei to the surrounding molecules (lattice). This is an exponential process, and the time required for 63% of the longitudinal magnetization, M_Z, to return to equilibrium is called the T1 relaxation time or spin–lattice relaxation time. The T1 relaxation time varies with different tissues and reflects the ability of their nuclei to transfer their excess energy to the surrounding molecules. Tissues with a high fluid content, such as cerebrospinal fluid (CSF), tend to have long T1 times because the high inherent energy of water inhibits the transfer of energy from excited hydrogen nuclei. Tissues with long T1 times produce low-intensity signals and appear dark in MR images. However, tissues with a high fat content, such as bone marrow, tend to have short T1 times that reflect the inherently low energy of fat and the relative ease with which energy is transferred from excited hydrogen nuclei. Tissues with short T1 times produce intense MR signals, displayed as bright white in a T1-weighted image.

When the RF pulse is applied, hydrogen nuclei precess around the Z-axis in phase (or in sync with each other). After the RF pulse is stopped, the magnetic moments of adjacent hydrogen nuclei begin to interfere with one another, causing the nuclei to dephase (i.e. to precess asynchronously relative to each other) with a resultant loss of the transverse magnetization, M_{XY}. The time constant that describes the exponential rate of loss of transverse magnetization is called the T2 relaxation time or the spin–spin relaxation time. As the transverse magnetization rapidly decays to zero, so does the amplitude and duration of the detected radio signal. T2 relaxation occurs more rapidly than T1 relaxation. Like T1 times, T2 times are also a feature of the tissues being examined. In fat tissues, the molecules are closely packed, and this results in more potent dephasing interactions between adjacent hydrogen nuclei. Thus, tissues with higher fat contents have short T2 relaxation times. A tissue with a short T1 time produces a low-intensity signal and is dark in the image. In contrast, the molecular arrangement of water is more widely spaced, and thus tissues containing more fluid have long T2 relaxation times. A tissue with long T2 produces a high-intensity signal and is bright in the image.

For every diagnostic task, the clinician must decide which imaging sequence will bring out the optimal image contrast. T1-weighted images are called 'fat images,' as fat has the shortest T1 relaxation time and the highest signal relative to other tissues and thus appears bright in this type of image. A high degree of anatomic detail is visible in this type of image because of its good image contrast. T1-weighted images are thus useful for depicting small anatomic regions, such as the TMJ, where high spatial resolution is needed.

T2-weighted images are called 'water images' because water has the longest T2 relaxation time and thus appears bright in the image. In general, the T2 times of abnormal tissues are longer than those of normal tissues. Images with T2 weighting are most commonly used when the practitioner is looking for inflammatory or other pathologic changes. Thus, T1-weighted images are most commonly used to demonstrate anatomy. In practice, images often must be acquired with both T1 and T2 weighting to separate the different tissues by contrast resolution.

5.4 The indications of MRI [3, 9]

1. Evaluating soft-tissue swellings of the head and neck regions
2. Evaluating benign and malignant neoplasms of the jaws and oral cavity in regard to soft-tissue extension
3. Determining the presence of malignant lymph node diseases or perineural invasion
4. Evaluating the position and integrity of the TMJ disk
5. Evaluating edematous changes in the fatty marrow as well as in the surrounding soft tissue
6. Evaluating salivary gland diseases including cysts, neoplasms, infections, and obstructions
7. Evaluating the course of the trigeminal nerve and the adjacent structures in trigeminal neuralgia cases
8. Identifying the location of the mandibular nerve
9. Midfield MRI for presurgical dental implant assessment

5.5 The advantages of MRI [3, 9]

1. MRI is a noninvasive and nonionizing imaging modality.
2. It offers the best resolution for tissues with low inherent contrast.
3. Contrast resolution—the imaging process differentiates adjacent soft tissues from one another. Further, if the RF pulse pattern is altered, the contrast between different tissues can be manipulated.
4. Multiplanar images can be obtained, including direct, sagittal, coronal, and oblique images.
5. Histopathologically acute and chronic phases and transit to fibrous phases can be simultaneously differentiated.
6. Artifacts associated with dental fillings or metal crowns are absent.
7. The high contrast level available in MRI makes the use of contrast agents unnecessary in most cases.
8. No adverse effects have been reported.

9. Manipulation of the image is possible.
10. Useful in determining the intramedullary spread.

5.6 The disadvantages of MRI [3, 9]

1. Claustrophobia: as the patient has to remain in a closed room within a large magnet for a long duration.
2. MRI apparatus is expensive to purchase, maintain, and operate
3. As the strong magnetic field used to image the patient is electrically and mechanically activated, MRI is not safe for patients with implants, cardiac pacemakers, implanted defibrillators, and prosthetic cardiac valves.
4. Metals such as surgical clips, aneurysm stents, etc. become distorted due to the magnetic field, so the MRI image becomes distorted
5. Signals are obtained only from the bone marrow; bone does not produce an MR signal.
6. The strong magnets used in MRI can be a serious threat to the placement of equipment even with advanced shielding.
7. The scanners used in MRI create a loud noise
8. MRI may not always differentiate between benign and malignant tumors or other disease processes.
9. Bone, teeth, air, and metallic objects all appear black, making differentiation difficult.

5.7 Safety concerns

Several incidents involving MR have been reported in ECRI Health Device Alerts (HDAs), U.S. Food and Drug Administration (FDA) Medical Device Reporting (MDR) [11]. The powerful magnetic field of the MR system attracts iron-containing (also known as ferromagnetic) objects and may cause them to move suddenly and with great force. This can pose a possible risk to the patient or anyone in an object's 'flight path.' The powerful magnetic field of the MR system will pull on any iron-containing object in the body. Every MRI facility has a comprehensive screening procedure and protocol that, when carefully followed, ensures that the MRI technologist and radiologist know about the presence of metallic implants and materials so that special precautions can be taken. The titanium, titanium alloy, and zirconia used in most dental implants are non-ferromagnetic metals, thus, it is safe to undergo MRI with these dental implants [12].

5.7.1 Contraindications for MRI [13]

(1) Vascular clips: a ferromagnetic vascular clip can raise concerns about MR-associated heating
(2) Foreign bodies: the shifting of metal foreign bodies under the influence of the magnetic field can damage vital structures and induce artifacts
(3) Coronary and peripheral arterial stents/aortic stent grafts cause artifacts, which can impair the evaluation of the stent itself

(4) Prosthetic heart valves and annuloplasty rings: minor interactions with the magnetic field
(5) Cardiac occluder devices/vena cava filters and embolization coils: these may induce occlusion of vessels when subjected to MRI
(6) Hemodynamic monitoring/support devices and temporary pacing devices: thermal injuries
(7) Permanent cardiac pacemakers, implantable defibrillators, and retained transvenous pacemakers
(8) Permanent contraceptive devices: heating and displacement
(9) Cochlear implants: force and torque induced by the magnetic field of the MRI represent hazards for the implant

Items that need to be removed before an MRI scan include the following [11]:

- Purses, wallets, credit cards, cards with magnetic strips
- Electronic devices such as beepers or cell phones
- Hearing aids
- Metal jewelry, watches
- Pens, paper clips, keys, coins
- Hair barrettes, hairpins
- Any article of clothing that has a metal zipper, buttons, snaps, hooks, underwires, or metallic threads Shoes, belt buckles, safety pins
- Makeup, nail polish, or other cosmetics that contain metallic particles

5.7.2 MRI and pregnancy

MRI is not considered hazardous to the fetus; however, a cautionary approach to MRI during pregnancy is recommended. MRI is indicated in pregnant women if other nonionizing forms of diagnostic imaging such as ultrasound are inadequate or if the examination provides more information that would otherwise require exposure to ionizing radiation such as x-rays or computed tomography [14].

In their large cohort study in Ontario, Canada, Ray *et al* concluded that 'MRI during the first trimester compared with non-exposure was not associated with increased risk of harm to the fetus or during early childhood.' However, gadolinium MRI at any time during pregnancy was associated with an increased risk of a broad set of rheumatological, inflammatory, or infiltrative skin conditions and with stillbirth or neonatal death [15].

5.8 Contrast agents

Injected contrast agents alter the intensity of the signal emitted by a tissue by altering the T1 or T2 relaxation times. Contrast enhancement is determined by the vascularity and the interstitial vascular space of the tissue involved.

Magnetic resonance contrast agents are classified as follows:

1. Ferromagnetic
2. Paramagnetic
3. Super magnetic

Paramagnetic contrast agents are the most popular and useful. The only paramagnetic agent is the lanthanide known as Gadolinium diethylene thiamine pantothenic acid (Gd-DTPA), which is most commonly used. Gadolinium (0.5 mol L^{-1}) is administered intravenously to improve tissue contrast. Gadolinium is not itself imaged but rather shortens the T1 and T2 relaxation times of the enhanced tissues, making them appear brighter. It also enhances some tumors by allowing them to be better differentiated from surrounding normal tissues.

Gadolinium does not contain iodine and therefore rarely causes an allergic reaction. However, there is evidence that gadolinium-based contrast media could be a cause of a debilitating disease called nephrogenic systemic fibrosis in some patients with renal dysfunction. Nephrogenic systemic fibrosis is characterized by skin thickening, hardening, and hyperpigmentation and disabling contractures in renal failure patients [16].

5.9 MRI interpretation

To describe the normal anatomy of the head and neck as depicted in MRI is beyond the scope of this text. Many textbooks are available that exclusively cover this aspect. In this section, we discuss various applications of MRI in dentistry for the evaluation of soft-tissue masses in the head and neck region, salivary gland imaging, the assessment of the TMJ articular disc and joint space, etc.

5.9.1 T1-weighted (T1W) images

These are called 'fat images,' as the fat appears bright in these images; they are more commonly used to demonstrate anatomy (Table 5.1).

Table 5.1. The appearances of various tissues and pathologies in T1-weighted images.

Hyperintense (very bright)	Isointense (bright/ intermediate)	Hypointense (gray/dark)
Fat	Organs	Water
Old blood	Muscle	Fibrous tissue
	Disk (TMJ)	Bone
		Fresh blood
		Air
Pathologies: 1. Hemorrhage 2. Cholesterol crystals 3. Fat 4. Lipomas 5. High-protein cysts (Thornwaldt's cyst, mucoceles, lymphoceles, hemorrhagic cysts of thyroid origin) 6. Hemorrhagic or highly calcified masses	1. Tumors 2. Ranulas 3. Parotid cysts 4. Chronic fungal disease 5. Adenitis	1. Lesions with dense calcification 2. Inflammatory lesions (edema) 3. Arteriovenous malformations 4. Mucous retention cysts 5. Acute fungal disease 6. Osteogenic or odontogenic masses 7. Sarcomas 8. Rhinoliths

Table 5.2. The appearances of various tissues and pathologies on T2-weighted images.

Hyperintense (very bright)	Isointense (bright/intermediate)	Hypointense (gray/dark)
Water	Fat Disk (TMJ)	Air Fibrous tissue Bone
Pathologies: 1. Inflammatory lesions 2. Acute sinusitis 3. Mucosal thickening 4. Abscesses 5. Cysts (ranulas, mucous retention cysts, thyroid cysts, branchial cleft cysts) 6. Benign masses (pleomorphic adenomas, polyps, lymph nodes, hemangiomas) 7. Synovial sarcomas 8. Adenoid cystic carcinomas	1. Most malignant lesions 2. Warthin's tumor 3. Oncocytomas 4. Adenocarcinomas 5. Squamous cell carcinoma 6. Schwannomas 7. Minor salivary gland tumors of the sinonasal cavity	1. Lesions with dense calcification 2. Fungal and actinomycotic infections, Rapidly flowing blood 3. Arteriovenous malformations 4. Aneurysms 5. Odontogenic masses, melanotic melanomas, amyloidomas 6. Fibromatous lesions, nodular fasciitis, aggressive fibromatosis, acutely hemorrhagic lesions, 7. Tornwaldt's cysts

5.9.2 T2-weighted (T2W) images

These are called 'water images,' as the water/fluid appears bright in these images. These images are more commonly used for identifying inflammatory or other pathologic changes (Table 5.2).

5.9.3 Soft-tissue lesions

MRI provides a soft-tissue window into the human body. In many instances, patients report with soft-tissue swellings with no inflammatory component or without any signs of inflammation. Conventional radiography fails to give information about the extent and content of the lesion. Computed tomography does not provide soft-tissue resolution to the same standard as MRI T1 and T2-weighted images. Thus, MRI is the best modality for the visualization of lesions such as lipomas, soft-tissue cysts, hemangiomas, and salivary gland imaging.

- *Lipoma*

A 49-year-old male patient reported with a swelling below the tongue on the right side that has been present for one year. On clinical examination, an ovoid swelling was noted over the right side of the floor of the mouth which had a smooth and shiny surface and well-defined edges. It was soft, non-fluctuant, non-compressible, non-reducible, and non-tender on palpation.

MRI showed a hyperintense signal on T1- and T2-weighted images with signal dropout on fat-suppressed sequences suggestive of a fat-containing lesion (figure 5.7).

• *Dermoid cyst*

A 29-year-old female patient reported with a swelling over the floor of the mouth that had caused slurred speech since childhood. The swelling showed a gradual increase in size to its current size over the last few years. On examination, a solitary swelling was seen over the floor of the mouth in the midline that had a smooth and intact overlying mucosa. On palpation, the swelling was soft and fluctuant, non-tender, compressible, and fixed to the underlying structures.

T1- and T2-weighted MRI revealed the presence of a well-defined, minimally hyperintense lesion exhibiting a fat fluid level within the lesion (figure 5.8).

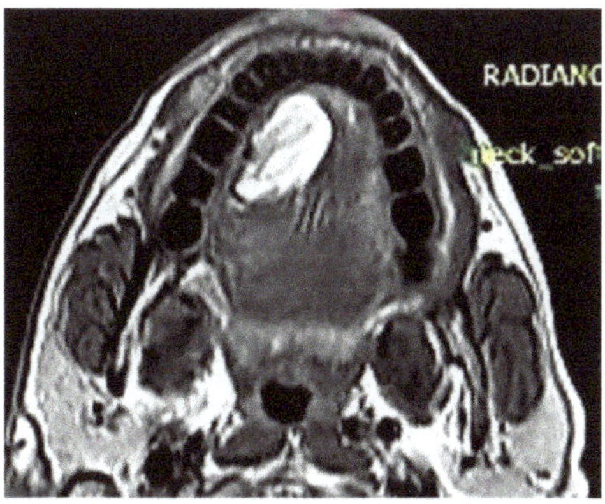

Figure 5.7a. Lipoma—An axial T1-weighted MRI image showing a well-defined hyperintense ovoid mass located at the right side of the floor of the mouth region.

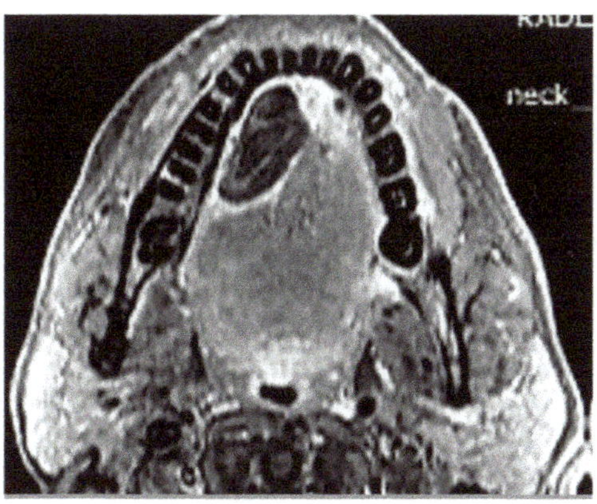

Figure 5.7b. Lipoma—An axial T1-weighted fat-suppression MRI image showing signal dropout in relation to the lesion on the right side of the floor of the mouth.

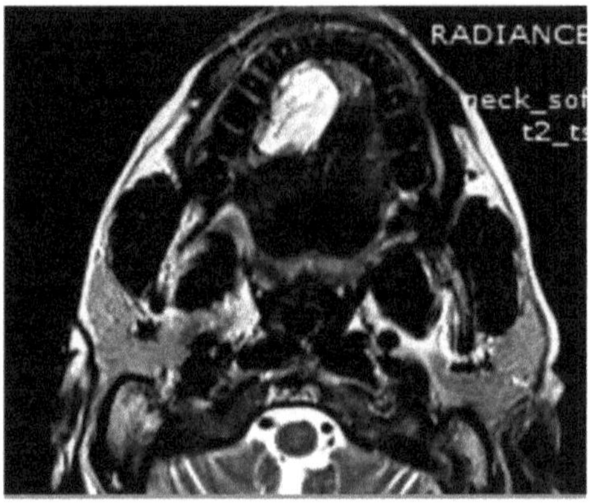

Figure 5.7c. Lipoma—An axial T2-weighted MRI image showing a hyperintense ovoid mass in relation to the right side of the floor of the mouth region.

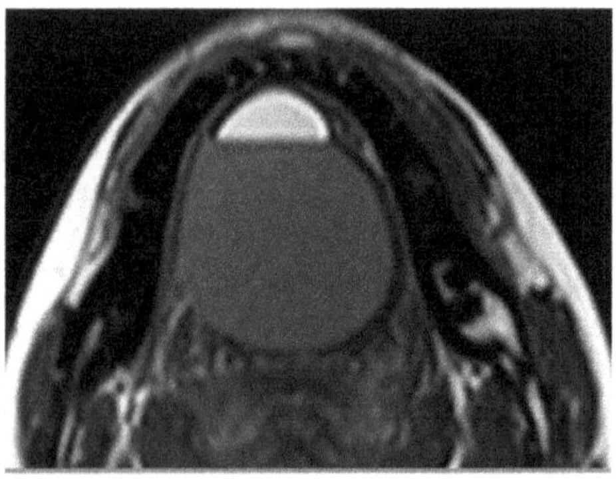

Figure 5.8a. Dermoid Cyst—an axial T1-weighted MRI of the floor of the mouth showing a midline, well-defined lesion that appeared minimally hyperintense with a fat fluid level within the lesion.

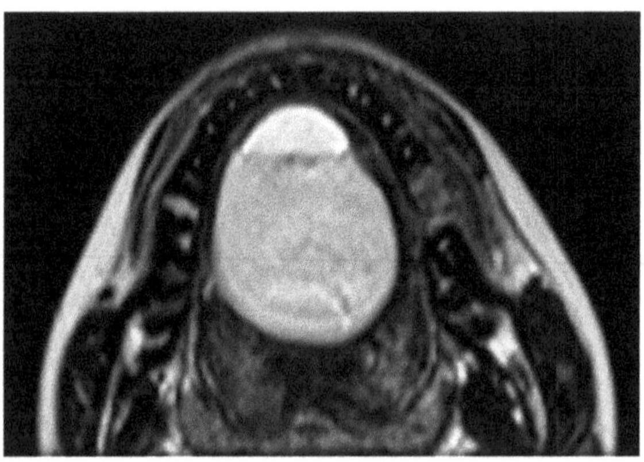

Figure 5.8b. Dermoid Cyst—an axial T2-weighted MRI of the floor of the mouth showing a hyperintense lesion with a fat fluid level.

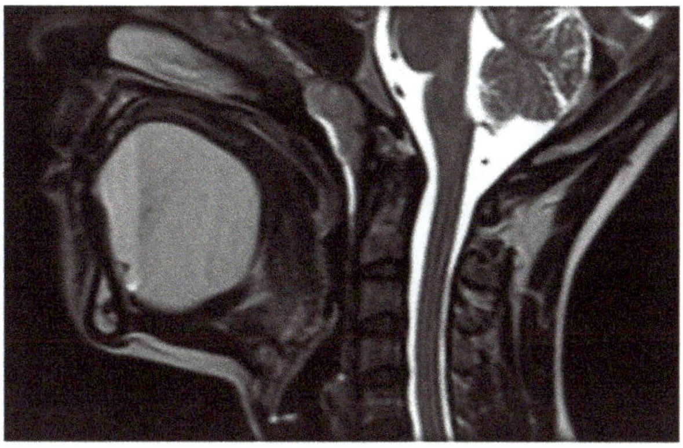

Figure 5.8c. Dermoid Cyst—a sagittal T2-weighted MRI of the floor of the mouth showing a hyperintense lesion with a fat fluid level.

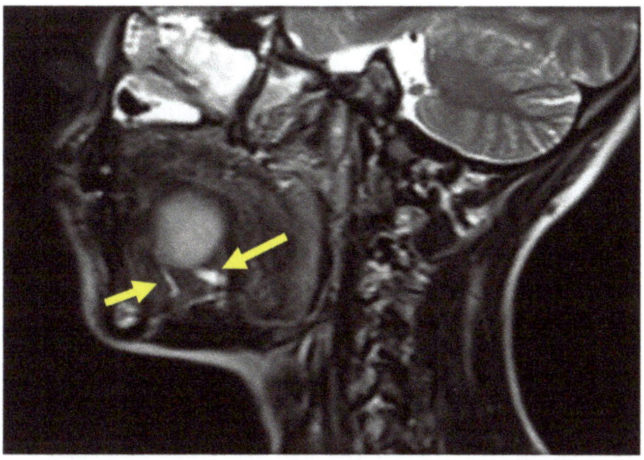

Figure 5.8d. Dermoid Cyst—a sagittal T2-weighted MRI of the floor of the mouth showing dilatation of the submandibular duct.

- *Intraparotid Cyst*

A 63-year-old male patient reported with pain and swelling along the lower jaw on the right side that had lasted for more than a month. On examination, a dome-shaped swelling with diffuse margins was noted over the right angle of the mandible. The skin over the swelling was intact and normal in appearance. Elevation of the left ear lobe was also noted. On palpation, the swelling was smooth and firm, mobile, non-compressible, and non-tender with no rise in local temperature.

MRI revealed the presence of a roughly ovoid mass along the inferomedial aspect of the right parotid gland. The lesion showed an intermediate intensity surrounded by a rim of low intensity on T1-weighted imaging and high signal intensity on T2-weighted imaging (figure 5.9).

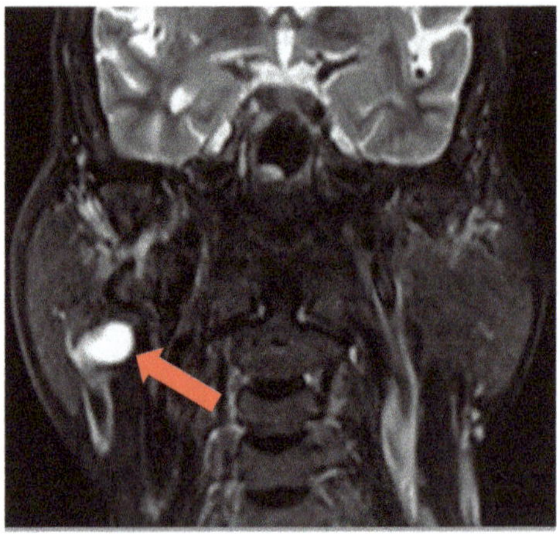

Figure 5.9a. Intraparotid cyst—a T1-weighted coronal view showing a heterogeneous roughly oval mass of intermediate intensity along the inferomedial aspect of the right parotid gland surrounded by a low-intensity rim.

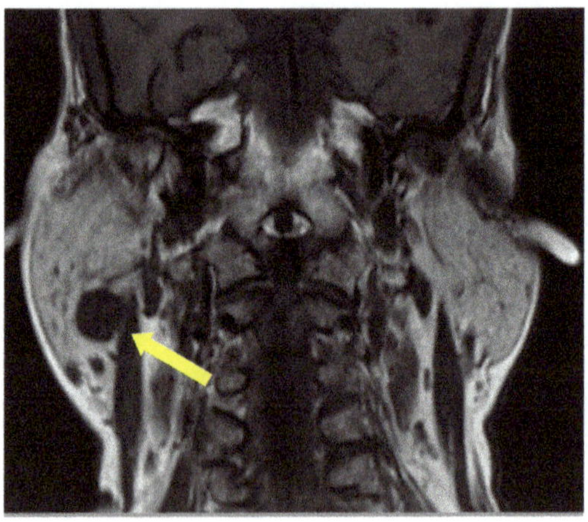

Figure 5.9b. Intraparotid cyst—a T2-weighted coronal view showing an oval-shaped mass of high intensity surrounded by a rim of low intensity.

5.10 Vascular lesions

- *Vascular malformation*

A 58-year-old female patient reported with a swelling over the floor of the mouth on right side that had been present for one month. On examination, an extraoral swelling was noted over the right submandibular and submental region with diffuse margins and normal appearance of the overlying skin. Intraorally, a diffuse swelling was noted over the floor of the mouth on the right side. Overlying mucosa showed the presence of distended blood vessels and elevation of the right Wharton's duct.

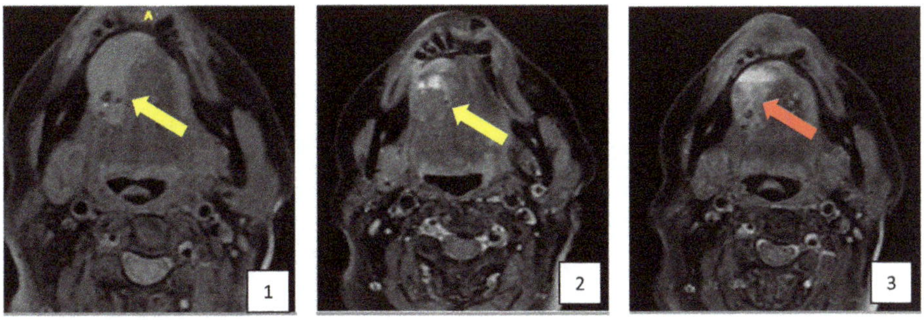

Figure 5.10. Sublingual hemangioma—T1-weighted MRI views of the floor of the mouth: (1) pre-contrast and (2) post-contrast showing homogeneous enhancement. (3) A post-contrast delayed axial T1-weighted MRI showing inhomogeneous enhancement of the lesion.

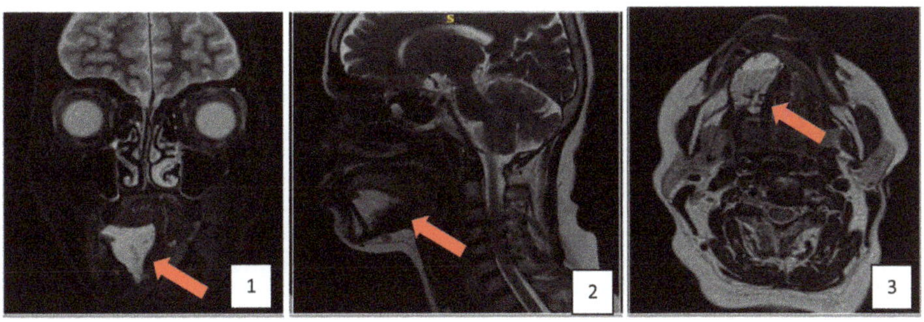

Figure 5.11. Sublingual hemangioma: (1) axial, (2) sagittal, and (3) coronal views: T2-weighted MRI showing a hyperintense lesion with a faint fluid level indenting the genioglossus muscle.

Plain MRI examination showed a well-demarcated lesion of abnormal signal intensity along the sublingual space on the right side indenting the genioglossus muscle. It was hyperintense on a T2-weighted sequence with a faint fluid level. A post-contrast MR image showed inhomogeneous enhancement of the lesion suggestive of a sublingual hemangioma (figures 5.10 and 5.11).

5.10.1 Salivary gland lesions

- *Pleomorphic adenoma of the parotid gland*

A 32-year-old female patient reported with pain over the region in front of her right ear that had been present for a year. On examination, no obvious swelling or asymmetry was noted; however, on palpation, a swelling soft to firm in consistency with tenderness to touch was encountered over the right pre-auricular region.

An MRI examination revealed the presence of a solid mass within the superficial lobe of the right parotid gland at the superior margin at the level of the right TMJ. It was isointense on a T1-weighted image and isointense to hyperintense on a T2-weighted image (figure 5.12).

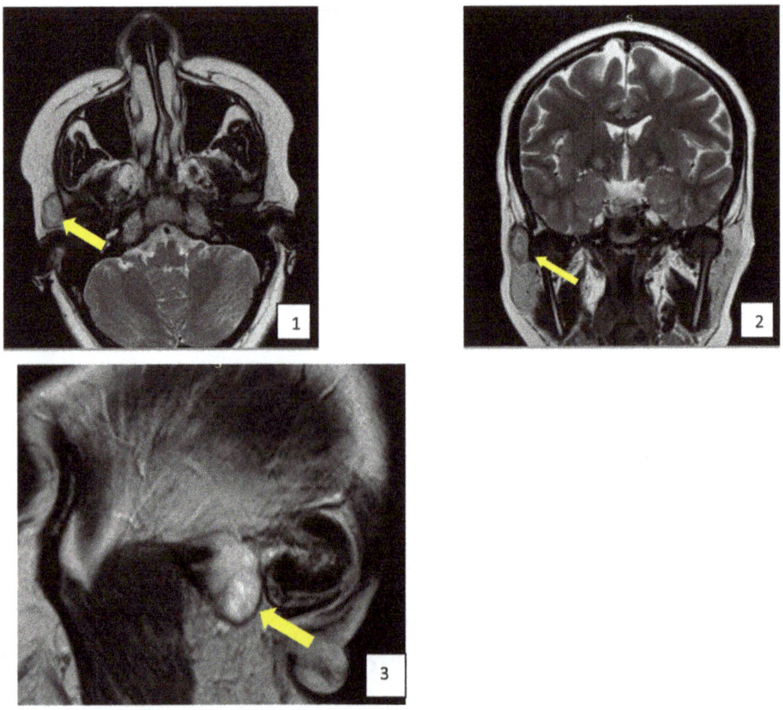

Figure 5.12. Pleomorphic adenoma: (1) axial, (2) coronal, and (3) sagittal views: T2-weighted MRI showing an isointense to hyperintense lesion within the superficial lobe of the right parotid gland.

- *Parotid sialolithiasis*

A 36-year-old male patient reported with the complaint of a swelling over the right side of the face that had been present for three days. There was a history of pain and an increase in the size of the swelling during meals. On clinical examination, a diffuse swelling was noted over the right pre-auricular region; the overlying skin appeared normal and intact. On palpation, the swelling was firm in consistency and non-tender. Intraorally, there was no evidence of swelling or any pathology.

MRI revealed a dilated right Stensen's duct with an 8 mm calculus seen within it (figure 5.13).

5.10.2 The temporomandibular joint

The TMJ is a special joint in its own way with a long list of disorders/pathologies. Most commonly, patients present with pain related to disc derangement with or without reduction. In such cases, MR imaging depends on the hydrogen nuclei content in the tissue as well as the tightness with which the hydrogen atoms are bound within molecules. The cortical outlines of the bone/condyle appear black in the MRI T1-weighted image, as the hydrogen atoms are tightly bound; they do not align themselves with the external magnetic field and thus do not produce a usable signal [9].

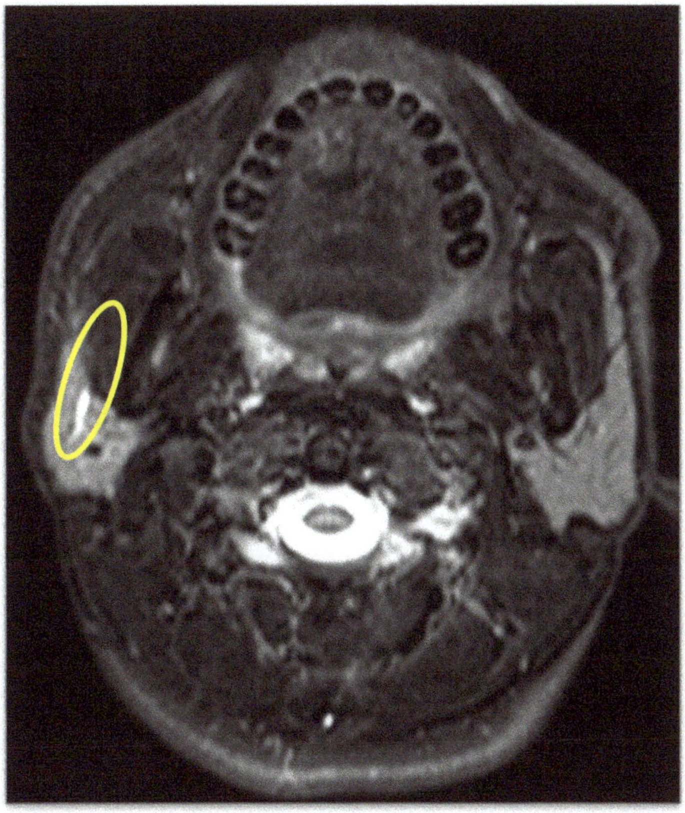

Figure 5.13. Parotid sialolithiasis—an axial section of a proton density weighted MRI showing a dilated right Stensen's duct with an 8?mm calculus seen within the duct at the anterior margin of the right parotid gland.

TMJ examination consists of both closed- and open-mouth views. Images are obtained in the oblique sagittal plane in a manner that orients the sections perpendicular to the condylar long axis. The T1- and T2-weighted sagittal MR images seen in figures 5.14(a)–(d) show a 'bow-tie' appearance of the articular disc in the closed- and open-mouth positions with respect to the head of the condyle. Coronal sections may be obtained to view the medial or lateral displacement of the disk.

The loosely bound hydrogen atoms such as in those in liquids or soft tissue tilt and align, producing a detectable signal in varying shades of gray. Hence, inflammatory changes, joint effusion, and hyperemia caused by increased vasculature in tissues can be detected in T2-weighted images [9].

- *Anterior disc displacement with reduction*

A 20-year-old male patient reported with a complaint of clicking from the left TMJ with a history of multiple episodes of locked jaw over a period of two years. On examination, mouth opening was within normal limits. Deviation of the mandible to the left was seen on mouth opening. Clicking in relation to the left

TMJ was also noted on mouth opening. Pain was experienced only on forceful mouth opening beyond the normal limits.

A T1-weighted MRI showed anterior displacement of the articular disc of the left TMJ in the closed-mouth position, which was seen to reduce to its normal position

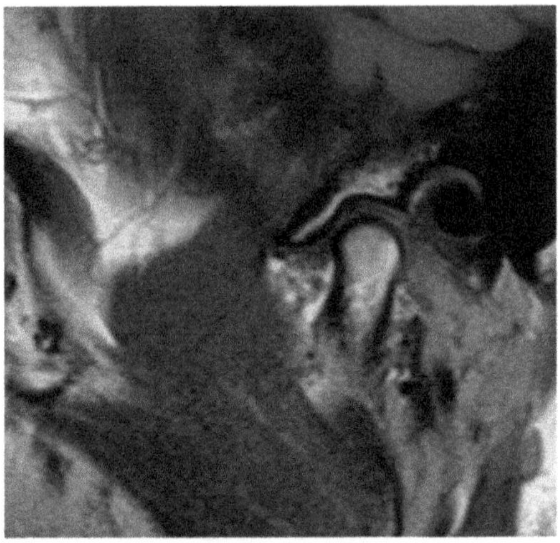

Figure 5.14a. A normal TMJ T1-weighted sagittal MR image (closed-mouth position) showing the articular disk with thick anterior and posterior bands and a thin intermediate zone,

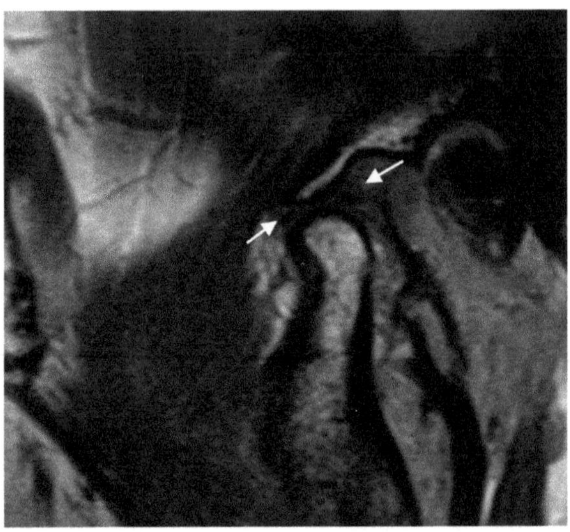

Figure 5.14b. A normal TMJ T1-weighted sagittal MR image (open-mouth position) showing the articular disk, which has a 'bow-tie' appearance.

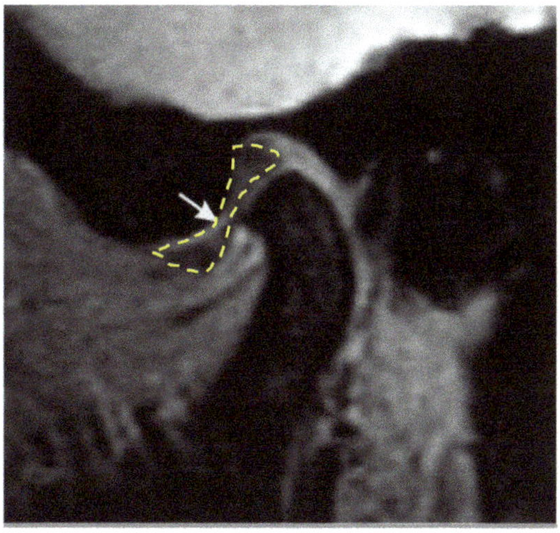

Figure 5.14c. A normal TMJ T2-weighted sagittal MR image (closed-mouth position) showing the articular disk with thick anterior and posterior bands and a thin intermediate zone (white arrow) creating a biconcave disk shape.

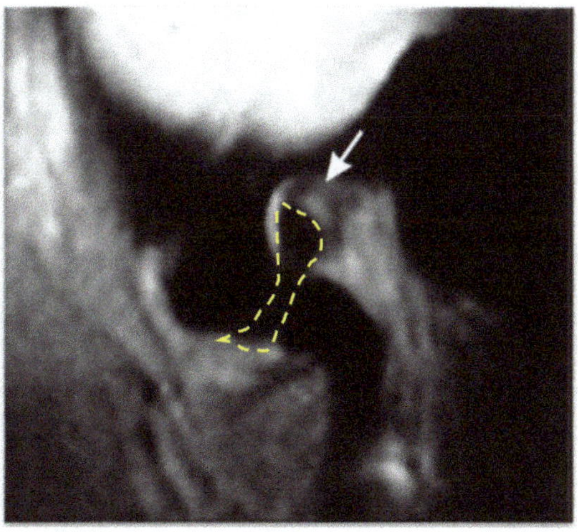

Figure 5.14d. A normal TMJ T2-weighted sagittal MR image (open-mouth position) showing the posterior band and retro-discal tissue (white arrow).

in the open-mouth view. It also showed thinning and sclerosis of the left mandibular condyle (figure 5.15).

- *Chronic osteomyelitis:*

A 36-year-old male patient reported with the complaint of reduced mouth opening with on and off swelling over the left side of lower jaw that had been present for a year. The swelling was not associated with pain. On clinical examination, a diffuse swelling was noted over the left masseter region. The overlying skin appeared

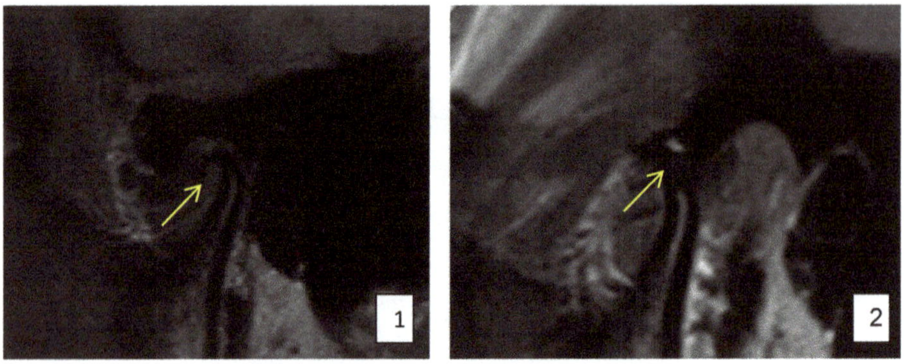

Figure 5.15. Anterior disc displacement with reduction. A T1-weighted MRI scan of the left TMJ sagittal section: (1) a closed-mouth view showing anterior displacement of the articular disc; (2) an open-mouth view showing reduction of the articular disc to its normal position.

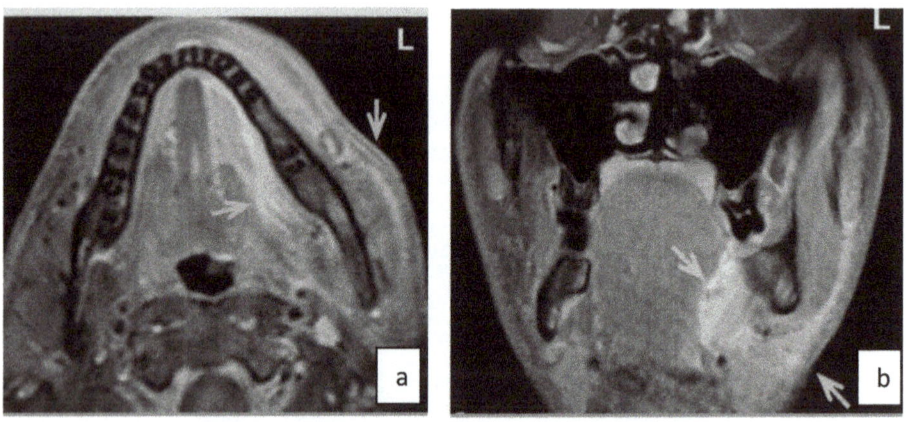

Figure 5.16. Chronic osteomyelitis. (a) An axial T2-weighted MR image showing a hyperintense left hemi-mandible. (b) A sagittal section showing enhancement in the surrounding musculature.

normal and intact, with no obvious foci of infection in the head and neck region. Mouth opening was restricted. The patient gave a history of swelling (space infection) in relation to a carious #38, which was treated four years previously. Contrast MRI showed a hyperintense left hemi-mandible with post-contrast enhancement in the surrounding musculature. Multiple enhanced enlarged lymph nodes were seen in the bilateral aspect. A probable diagnosis of chronic sclerosing osteomyelitis was given (figure 5.16).

5.10.3 Trigeminal neuralgia

Trigeminal neuralgia (TN) is primarily diagnosed based on the patient's history and clinical findings. Recently, MRI has been playing an essential role in confirming TN diagnoses and at times differentiating them from other orofacial pain cases.

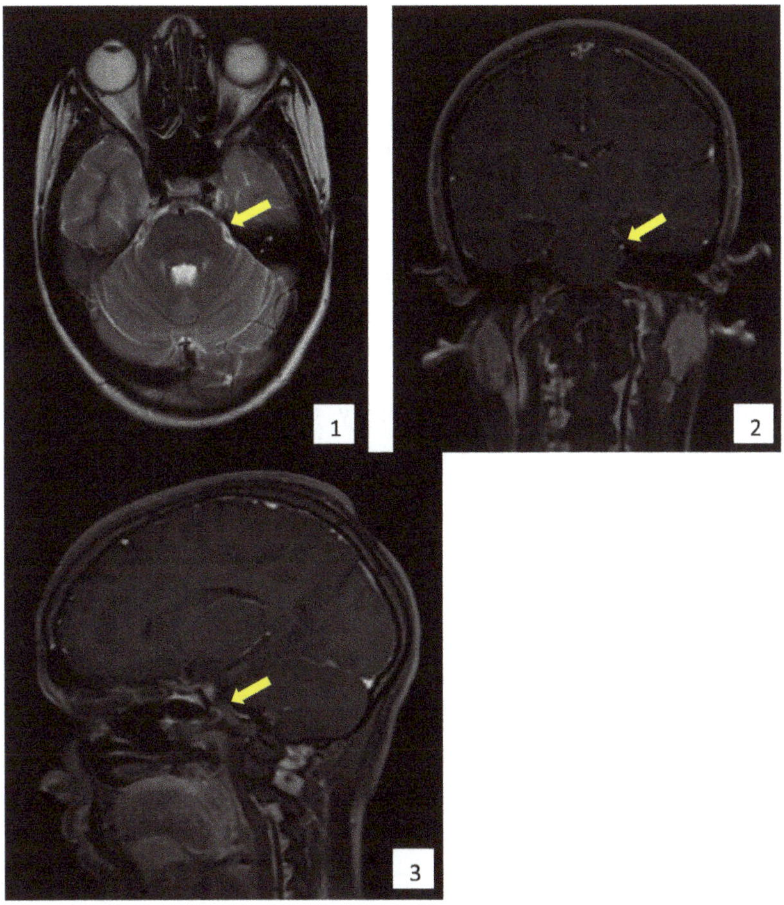

Figure 5.17. T2-weighted images: (1) axial, (2) coronal, and (3) sagittal views showing thickening and subtle enhancement of the left trigeminal nerve.

A 21-year-old female patient reported with pain over the left side of the face on touching the face. The pain was sharp and shooting in nature; it was episodic and lasted for about 1 min. The patient described it as 'electric shock—like pain.' It involved the left temporal, orbital, and malar regions.

MRI T2-weighted images showed thickening and subtle enhancement of the left trigeminal nerve suggesting a neurogenic tumor (figure 5.17).

5.11 Conclusions

MRI is a complex but effective diagnostic modality that offers the most sensitive and noninvasive approach for imaging. It has a variety of clinical applications in the field of medical diagnosis, staging, and follow-up of disease. This chapter gives an insight into the appropriate utilization of MRI along with case scenarios to highlight its importance in diagnosing routinely encountered oral and maxillofacial pathologies.

With newer pulse sequences and advances, MRI has definitely benefited the world at large by enabling physicians as well as patients to gain a clear and a better understanding of various diseases and disorders. But with advancing technology and improvised equipment comes the responsibility of taking wise decisions and making judicious use of the same, which should be borne in mind by both clinicians and imaging centers.

Acknowledgments

The case scenarios and MRI images are included in the chapter courtesy of the Department of Oral Medicine and Radiology, Goa Dental College and Hospital, Bambolim, Goa. Figures 5.1–5.6 were drawn by Dr Aniket Vaidya, lecturer in the Department of Oral Medicine and Radiology, Goa Dental College and Hospital, Bambolim, Goa.

References

[1] Beckmann N M, West O C, Nunez Jr D, Kirsch C F, Aulino J M, Broder J S, Cassidy R C, Czuczman G J, Demertzis J L, Johnson M M and Motamedi K 2019 ACR appropriateness criteria suspected spine *trauma. J. Am. Coll. Radiol.* **16** S264–85

[2] American College of Radiology Glossary of MRI Terms https://www.acr.org/-/media/ACR/files/radiology-safety/MR-safety/MRGlossary.pdf

[3] Katti G, Ara S A and Shireen A 2011 Magnetic resonance imaging (MRI)—a review *Int. J. Dent. Clin.* **3** 65–70

[4] Scherzinger A L and Hendee W R 1985 Basic principles of magnetic resonance imaging—an update, in high-tech medicine [special issue] *West J. Med* **143** 782–92

[5] Sobol W T 2012 Recent advances in MRI technology: implications for image quality and patient safety *Saudi J. Ophthalmol.* **26** 393–99

[6] Geva T 2006 Magnetic resonance imaging: historical perspective *J. Cardiovasc. Magn. Reson.* **8** 573–80

[7] Westbrook C, Roth C K and Talbot J 2011 *MRI in Practice* 4th edn (London: Wiley)

[8] Muhammed I 2014 An overview on MRI physics and its clinical applications *Int. J. Current Pharmaceutical and Clinical Research* **4** 185–93

[9] Mallya S and Lam E 2018 Other imaging modalities *White and Pharoah's Oral Radiology* 8th edn (Amsterdam: Elsevier) 13 541–59

[10] Lakrimi M *et al* 2011 The principles and evolution of magnetic resonance imaging *J. Phys. Conf. Ser.* **286** 012016

[11] Ng K H, Ahmad A C, Nizam M, Abdullah B 2003 Magnetic resonance imaging: Health effects and safety *Proceedings of the International Conference on Non-Ionizing Radiation at UNITEN (ICNIR2003) Electromagnetic Fields and Our Health* pp 1–15

[12] Hoque M E *et al* 2022 Titanium and titanium alloys in dentistry: current trends, recent developments, and future prospects *Heliyon* **8** e11300

[13] Dill T 2008 Contraindications to magnetic resonance imaging: non-invasive imaging *Heart* **94** 943–8

[14] Shellock F G and Crues J V 2004 MR procedures: biologic effects, safety, and patient care *Radiology* **232** 635–52

[15] Ray J G *et al* 2016 Association between MRI exposure during pregnancy and fetal and childhood outcomes *JAMA* **316** 952–61

[16] Pan D *et al* 2011 Manganese-based MRI contrast agents: past, present and future *Tetrahedron* **67** 8431–44

Chapter 6

Radiography as a diagnostic tool for oral hard-tissue diseases

Amir I O Ibrahim and Desigar Moodley

6.1 Introduction

Oral diseases can be classified as diseases of the soft or hard tissues. The diagnosis of such diseases is a complex procedure that requires the use of multiple diagnostic tools. Radiography plays an essential role in the diagnosis of such diseases, especially hard-tissue diseases. Numerous dental radiographs and radiographic techniques are used, such as conventional radiography, digital radiography, and cone beam computed tomography. In this chapter, we discuss the roles of the different radiographs used for the diagnosis of oral hard-tissue diseases in detail.

6.2 The history and physics of x-rays

On 8 November 1895, Wilhelm Conrad Röntgen discovered a new type of radiation. This discovery occurred after a series of experiments in which he was investigating the phenomenon of electrical discharge across rarefied gases (Robotti 2013). During his experiments, Dr Röntgen discovered that a fluorescent screen became bright when brought into close contact with a highly evacuated tube connected to a large induction coil in a dark room. He concluded that the fluorescence of the screen was the result of invisible rays, which were later termed x-rays. He also concluded that these invisible rays (x-rays) possess the following properties:

1. They are emitted when the cathode ray collides with the tube wall.
2. These rays are transmitted in a straight line without reflection or refraction.
3. They have the ability to penetrate different surfaces.
4. They can be detected by a photographic plate.

The x-ray was then defined as an electromagnetic type of radiation characterized by continuous cyclic waves of combined electrical and magnetic fields (Seibert 2004). The mechanism of x-ray production requires the emission of electrons from the

doi:10.1088/978-0-7503-5316-8ch6

cathode (filament) of a heated tube. The tube is heated by applying a high voltage between the cathode and an anode. The emitted electrons are deposited on the anode (target), which is usually tungsten, molybdenum, or rhodium. As a result of the electrons hitting the target, the kinetic energy of the electrons is converted into heat and x-rays (Seibert 2004, Yue *et al* 2002).

Furthermore, x-ray tubes can produce photons when either the electrical current (measured in milliamperes (mA)) or the voltage (measured in kilovolts (kV)) of the x-ray tube is altered. The electrical current determines the number of electrons released from the cathode to the anode. When the electrical current is increased, the number of released electrons is increased, and thus a large number of photons is produced by the x-ray tube. Altering the voltage can affect the velocity of the released electrons, which has a direct relationship with the energy of the photons released by an x-ray tube (McCollough 1997).

In the dental field, several dentists attempted to use x-rays as an adjunct diagnostic tool in dentistry after they were first discovered. The first dental radiograph was made by Dr Otto Walkhoff, a German dentist, in 1985. Dr Walkhoff placed a glass photographic plate wrapped in black paper and rubber in his mouth and exposed himself to 25 min of x-rays. During the same period, an American physician, Dr W J Morton, made the first skull radiograph and demonstrated the advantages of x-rays in dentistry. Following these experiments, several dentists experimented with the role of x-rays in dental practice by conducting different experiments in the oral cavity. Unfortunately, many of those dental researchers died from radiation overexposure (Iannucci and Howerton 2021, Langland and Langlais 1995).

6.3 X-ray–tissue interactions

One of the main roles of x-rays is to aid in the diagnosis of hard or soft tissue diseases by capturing a picture or shadow of the tissue that is subjected to x-rays in a receptor (x-ray film). To understand how an object (hard or soft tissue) appears on a receptor, an understanding of how x-rays interact with tissues is essential.

The production of an x-ray image (radiograph) usually results from the interaction of the x-ray beam with the human tissues (hard or soft). Different tissues react differently when exposed to an x-ray beam. This interaction results in a variable degree of x-ray transmission through different human tissues, producing a superimposed shadow of the human tissue. The transmitted fraction is then captured by an x-ray detector and converted into an image (Seibert 2004).

6.4 The oral environment

The oral cavity represents the first part of the digestive system. It consists of soft and hard tissues. The soft tissue includes the tongue, the gingiva, the oral mucosa, the soft palate, and the floor of the mouth. The hard tissue includes the teeth with their surrounding alveolar bone (figure 6.1).

The functions of the oral cavity include mastication, speech, and facilitating swallowing. Furthermore, the oral cavity acts as a habitat for different microbial

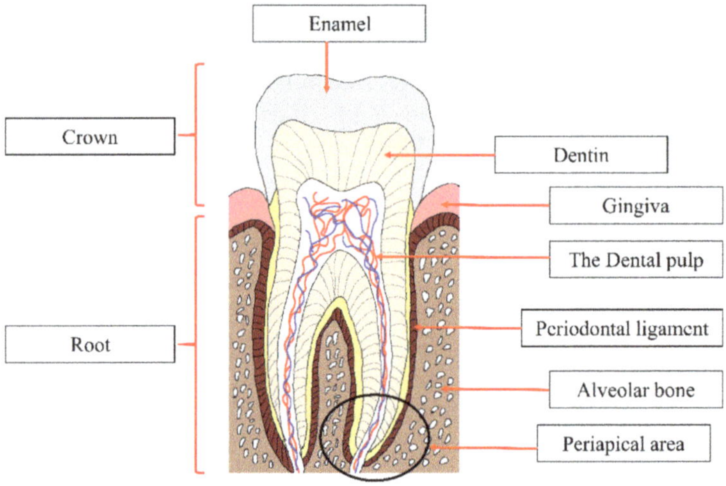

Figure 6.1. The dental hard tissue showing the tooth parts with the surrounding alveolar bone and periapical area.

species (normal flora), including bacteria, fungi, and viruses, which represent the normal flora of the oral cavity. More than 700 microbial species have been identified in the oral cavity (Aas *et al* 2005, Paster *et al* 2006), attached to different parts of the oral cavity in a structure known as dental plaque (Hardie 1992). The research literature shows that most dental hard-tissue diseases (dental caries and periodontal diseases) are associated with microbial infection from this oral microbial flora (Berezow and Darveau 2011, Chen *et al* 2020, Eidt *et al* 2020, Socransky 1970, Tanzer *et al* 2001).

Radiographs are among the most important tools for the diagnosis of dental hard-tissue diseases. The availability of high-quality radiographs is essential for a proper and accurate diagnosis of such diseases, as they can detect hidden lesions that are not seen clinically. Therefore, dental radiographic techniques and equipment have shown progressive improvement in meeting the need to diagnose dental diseases.

6.5 Radiographs as a diagnostic tool for oral diseases

The use of dental radiology plays an important role in the diagnosis of oral diseases (hard and soft tissue). The discovery of x-rays facilitated a better understanding of oral disease progress, and, at the same time, aided in the diagnosis of dental hard-tissue diseases such as dental caries, periodontal diseases, and the detection of alveolar bone fracture lines. In addition, dental radiology allows dentists to observe the progress of dental development and detect the presence of any dental developmental anomalies. Furthermore, the use of other radiological techniques, such as MRI, can assist in the diagnosis of oral soft tissue diseases. The following section discusses the role of different radiographs in the diagnosis of oral hard-tissue diseases only.

6.6 The role of radiology in the diagnosis of dental hard-tissue diseases

Dental hard-tissue diseases are diseases that involve the destruction of the mineralized dental tissue, such as enamel, dentin, and cementum. In addition, they involve the destruction of the supporting alveolar bone, which results in periodontal diseases (figure 6.2). Such destruction is mainly caused by the acid produced by the oral microflora. This acid results in the demineralization of the hard tissue by removing some minerals, such as hydroxyapatite.

One of the most prevalent oral hard-tissue diseases worldwide is dental caries, which is defined as 'a biofilm-mediated, diet-modulated, multifactorial, non-communicable, dynamic disease resulting in net mineral loss of dental hard tissues' (Machiulskiene *et al* 2020). The prevalence of dental caries ranges from 25% in some countries, such as Australia, to as much as 99% in other countries, such as South Africa (Chan *et al* 2021). Other studies have found that the prevalence of dental caries ranges from 46.2% in children to 53% in adults (Kazeminia *et al* 2020). The pathogenesis of dental caries starts with the fermentation of remnants of carbohydrates in the oral cavity by some oral microorganisms. This fermentation process results in a dramatic decrease in the pH of the oral environment, especially in the first 30 min after carbohydrate consumption (Bowen 2013). The radical drop in pH, together with the acid produced by the oral microorganisms, result in the removal of minerals (demineralization) such as hydroxyapatite from the tooth surface and eventually the loss of tooth structure (enamel, dentin, or cementum), depending on the progression of the caries process (Featherstone 2008).

The progression of dental caries can be detected (diagnosed) clinically (visually) or radiographically (Abogazalah and Ando 2017). The use of radiographs plays an important role in caries detection and supports clinical diagnosis. The basic principle of using a radiograph in the detection of dental caries is based on changes in the radiographic density in different parts of the tooth structure as a result of reduced mineral content in the carious part of the tooth structure compared to its sound

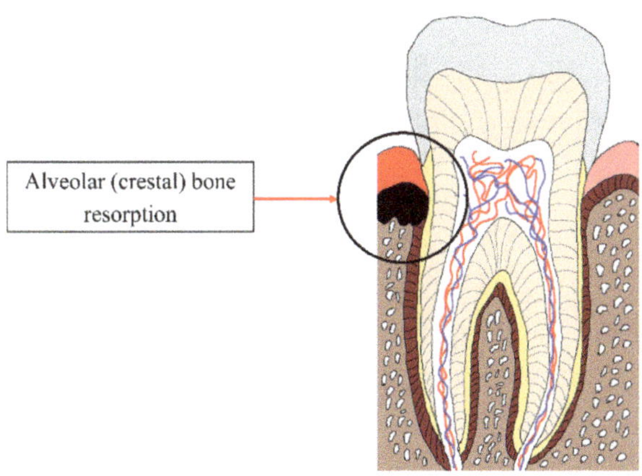

Figure 6.2. Alveolar (crestal) bone destruction indicating periodontal diseases.

structure. Radiographs with higher density may indicate the presence of dental caries in the imaged area. Furthermore, the radiographic detection of carious lesions requires one half or one third of a sound tooth structure to be affected by carious lesions (Dove 2001). Different radiographic parameters may affect the accuracy of caries detection performed using radiography, such as:

1. The x-ray exposure parameters
2. The type of x-ray receptor used
3. The x-ray image processing technique
4. The display system.
5. The viewing conditions
6. The training and experience of the observer

As the carious lesion extends apically toward the dental pulp, inflammation of the pulp tissue starts, resulting in pulpitis. As caries progress, microbial invasion of the pulp tissue space starts, causing inflammation and eventually necrosis of the pulp tissue. Pulp inflammation and microbial invasion can progress further apically into the periapical tissue area, resulting in the destruction of the mineralized tissue around the apex and hence the name apical periodontitis (figure 6.3) (inflammation of the tissue around the apex of the tooth) (Zero *et al* 2011).

Taken together, pulp and periapical diseases are known as endodontic diseases. The use of x-rays in endodontics is essential for the diagnosis of pulp and periapical disease, the assessment of treatment difficulty during treatment (root canal cleaning), and the evaluation of post-treatment healing. Different radiographic images with different views can be used; however, periapical radiographs and, more recently, cone beam computed tomography are the most commonly used types of radiographic image (Setzer and Lee 2021). The full details of these radiographic techniques will be discussed later in this chapter.

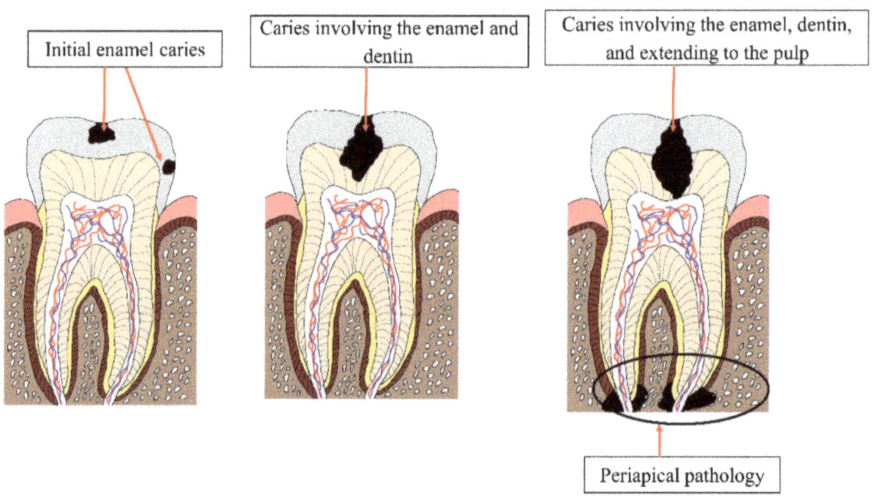

Figure 6.3. The progression of dental caries.

Periodontal diseases are diseases that involve a wide variety of chronic inflammatory conditions of the soft and hard tissues that surround and support the teeth. Such tissues include the gingiva, alveolar mucosa, periodontal ligament, and alveolar bone (Pihlstrom *et al* 2005). The etiology of periodontal diseases is mainly microbial toxins that result from plaque accumulation and retention around the periodontal tissue. The management of periodontal disease is based on the degree of periodontal destruction. Radiographs play an important role in determining the degree of periodontal destruction (alveolar bone) and hence proper treatment. Various radiographs with different views can be used in order to identify the amount of alveolar bone loss, the type of alveolar bone loss (vertical or horizontal), the presence of anatomical defects around the tooth that may enhance plaque retention, and the presence of overhang restoration around the tooth (Tugnait *et al* 2000).

6.7 Dental radiography

Dental radiographs can be classified into either intraoral radiography or extraoral radiography. The main difference between the two types is related to the location of the x-ray film (receptor). When the x-ray receptor is placed intraorally, the name used is intraoral radiographs. However, in the case of extraoral radiographs, the x-ray receptor is placed extraorally and hence the name used is extraoral radiographs. Different types of intraoral and extraoral radiographs are listed in table 6.1.

Table 6.1. Different types of dental radiographs based on the location of the x-ray film.

Intraoral radiographs	*Extraoral radiographs*
Periapical	Panoramic
Bitewing	Lateral jaw
Occlusal	Lateral cephalometric
	Posteroanterior
	Waters
	Submentovertex
	Reverse town
	Transcranial
	Tomographic projection

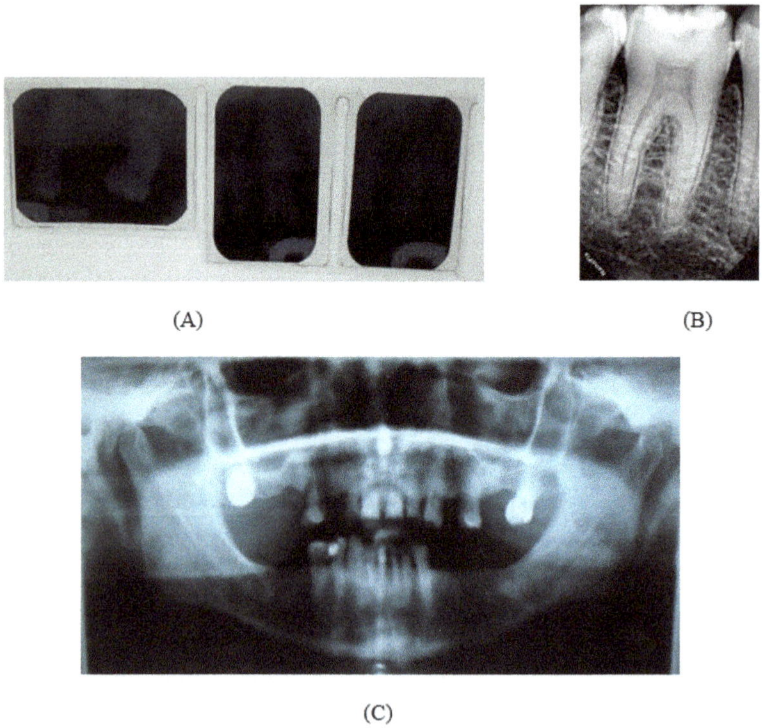

Figure 6.4. Different types of dental radiograph: (A) and (C) conventional radiographs, (B) a digital radiograph. Courtesy of the Dental Clinic Complex, College of Dentistry, King Faisal University.

Furthermore, as a result of the introduction of the digital dentistry concept, another classification has been developed, which contains two types of dental radiography: (i) conventional radiography, which uses dental film to capture x-ray images; (ii) digital radiography, which uses software to process the x-ray images (figure 6.4). Digital radiographs are further discussed later in this chapter. This chapter is limited to discussing the types of radiographs that are routinely used for the diagnosis of dental hard-tissue diseases.

6.7.1 Periapical radiographs

The periapical radiograph is an intraoral radiograph in which the x-ray film (receptor) is placed inside the oral cavity. This type of x-ray allows visualization of the entire tooth with the surrounding periapical area, hence the name periapical radiograph (figure 6.5).

The periapical radiograph is one of the types of intraoral radiograph most commonly used during a routine dental examination, as it provides information regarding the presence of dental caries, the presence of any lesion around the periapical area, the presence of periodontal diseases, and the presence or absence of fracture within the tooth (crown or root) and its surrounding bone (Bourguignon *et al* 2020, Corbet *et al* 2009, Dayo *et al* 2021).

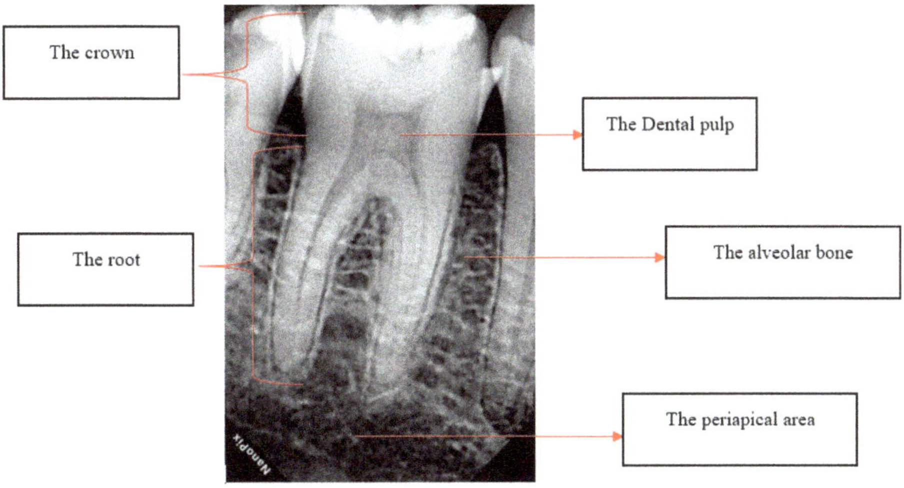

Figure 6.5. A periapical radiograph showing the tooth crown, root, and periapical area. Courtesy of the Dental Clinic Complex, College of Dentistry, King Faisal University.

A periapical radiograph can be obtained through the use of two techniques, namely the paralleling technique and the bisecting angle technique (figure 6.6). The paralleling technique involves the placement of the x-ray film (receptor) parallel to the tooth, with the x-ray beam running perpendicular to the x-ray film. This is controlled by the use of an x-ray holder (beam alignment device) (figure 6.7). However, in the bisecting technique, the x-ray film is placed on the lingual surface of the tooth being radiographed. The x-ray beam runs perpendicular to an imaginary line that divides the two lines; one runs parallel to the long axis of the tooth, and another line runs parallel to the x-ray film (receptor) (Setzer and Lee 2021).

The use of the paralleling technique produces more accurate image geometry (tooth length, alveolar bone level) compared to the bisecting technique (figure 6.8). Furthermore, the presence of proximal caries can be detected better in the paralleling technique than in the bisecting technique. In addition, a reproducible image can easily be obtained in the case of the paralleling technique, as a beam alignment device is always used to direct the x-ray beam to the same angle as the receptor (Gupta *et al* 2014).

The periapical radiograph is one of the most common radiographic images used for the diagnosis of dental caries, as it shows the full length of the tooth with the surrounding 2 mm of the periapical region (Prados-Privado *et al* 2020) (figure 6.5). However, it has a limited role in the detection of small carious lesions that are located in the buccal or lingual surface of the tooth structure. This results from the superimposition of sound tooth structure on the carious lesion. This superimposition is the result of the nature of the periapical radiograph, which shows only two dimensions of a three-dimensional object (figure 6.9).

Similarly, the detection of an initial proximal carious lesion may be difficult from a periapical view unless one half to one third of the sound tooth structure is affected

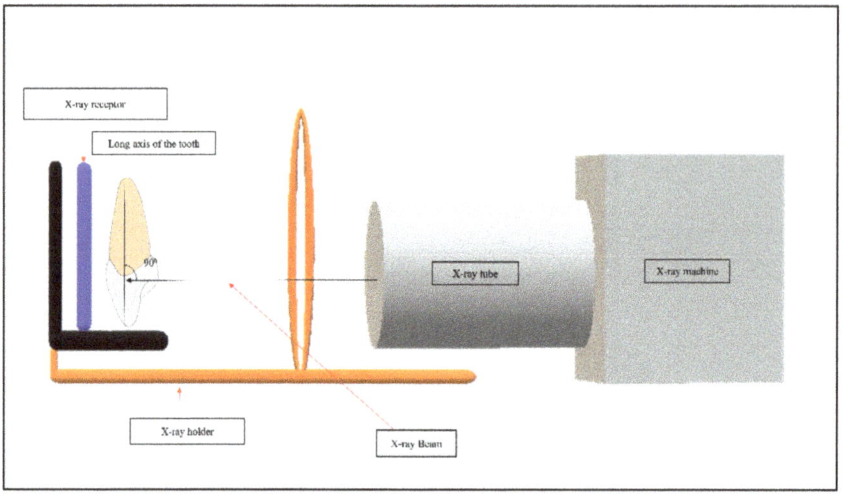

(A)

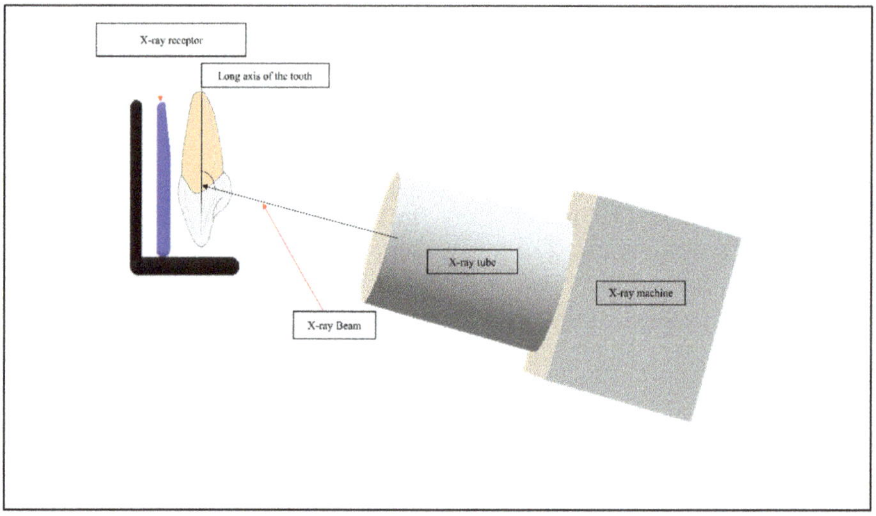

(B)

Figure 6.6. Periapical radiograph techniques: (A) the paralleling technique and (B) the bisecting technique.

(demineralized) by a carious lesion, and hence different radiographic views may be suggested, such as the bitewing radiograph (figure 6.10).

The periapical radiograph has an essential role in the diagnosis of endodontic diseases (before treatment), during treatment, and in evaluating the healing of the periapical tissue following root canal treatment. Before any endodontic treatment is started, a periapical radiograph may provide information such as the preoperative status of the periapical area, an evaluation of the anatomical complexity of the root canal system, an evaluation of the length of the root, and the presence of

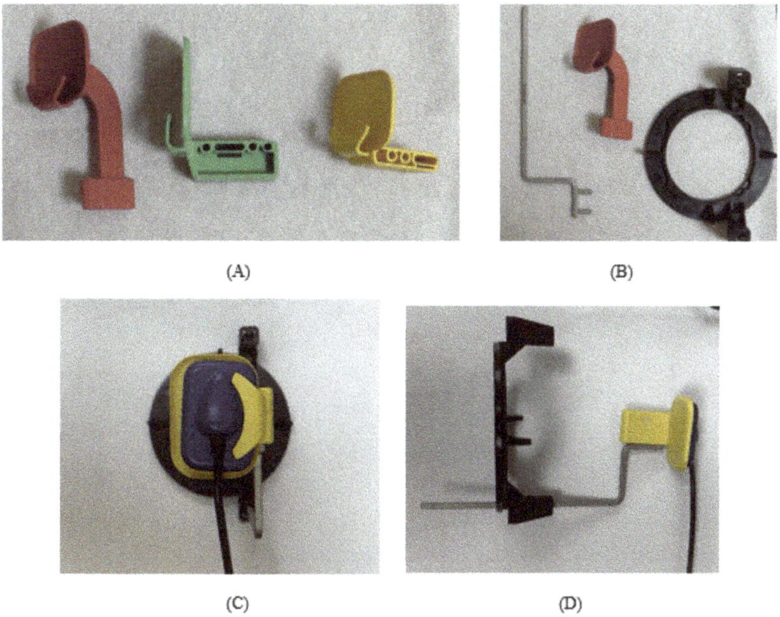

Figure 6.7. Different types of x-ray holder: (A), (B) beam alignment devices and (C) and (D) assembled devices.

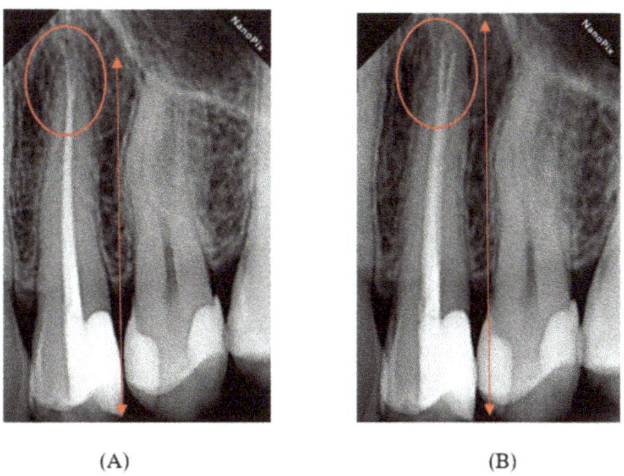

Figure 6.8. Periapical radiograph captured using (A) the paralleling technique, (B) the bisecting technique. The tooth appears elongated when the bisecting technique (B) is used. In addition, the presence of two root canals at the root apex is visible in the bisecting view. Courtesy of the Dental Clinic Complex, College of Dentistry, King Faisal University.

calcification within the root canal system (figure 6.11). Furthermore, one of the requirements of radiographic images for endodontic treatment is to obtain a reproducible x-ray image. The use of paralleling periapical radiographs may allow reproducible x-ray images to be captured (Patel *et al* 2009).

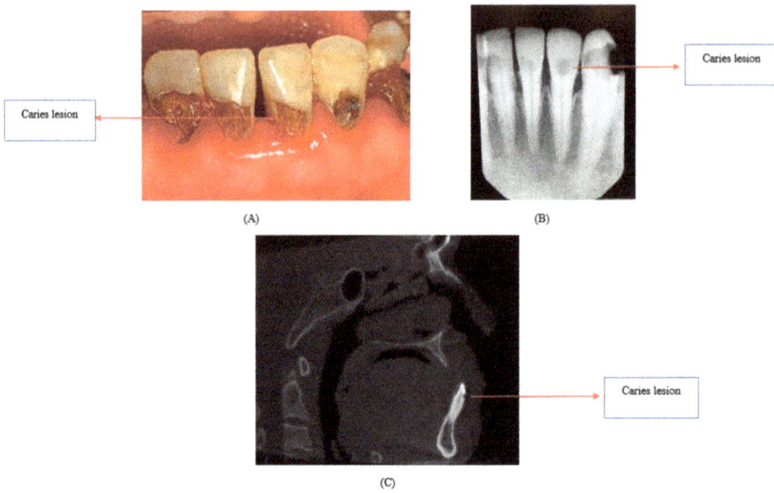

Figure 6.9. A carious lesion is observed on the labial surface of the central incisors (A). Periapical radiograph showing a radiolucent area in the labial surface of the central incisors (B), (the depth of the carious lesion cannot be determined), Cone beam computed tomography showing the depth of the carious lesion (C). Courtesy of the Dental Clinic Complex, College of Dentistry, King Faisal University.

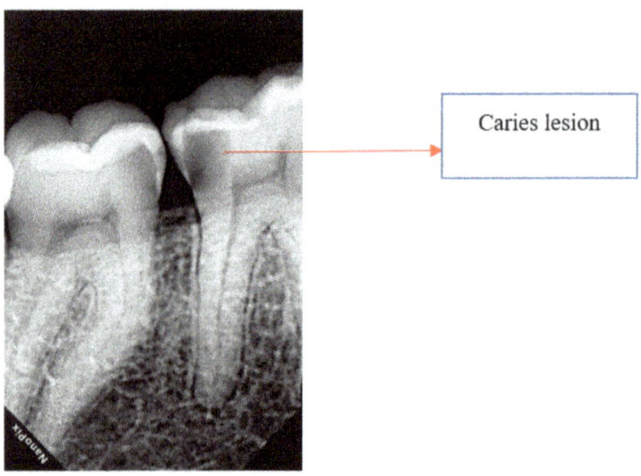

Figure 6.10. A periapical radiograph showing a proximal caries lesion. Notice that the caries lesion involves more than one third of the sound tooth structure. Courtesy of the Dental Clinic Complex, College of Dentistry, King Faisal University.

Although periapical radiographs are still used during routine endodontic investigations, some shortcomings of this radiographic view have been observed, such as:

1. The two-dimensional view of a three-dimensional object captured by the periapical radiograph may require multiple exposures (radiographic images) at different angulations in order to visualize the tooth from different angles (Velvart *et al* 2001).
2. The difficulty in obtaining the accurate anatomy of the tooth as a result of a geometrical alteration (over-angulated or down-angulated images).

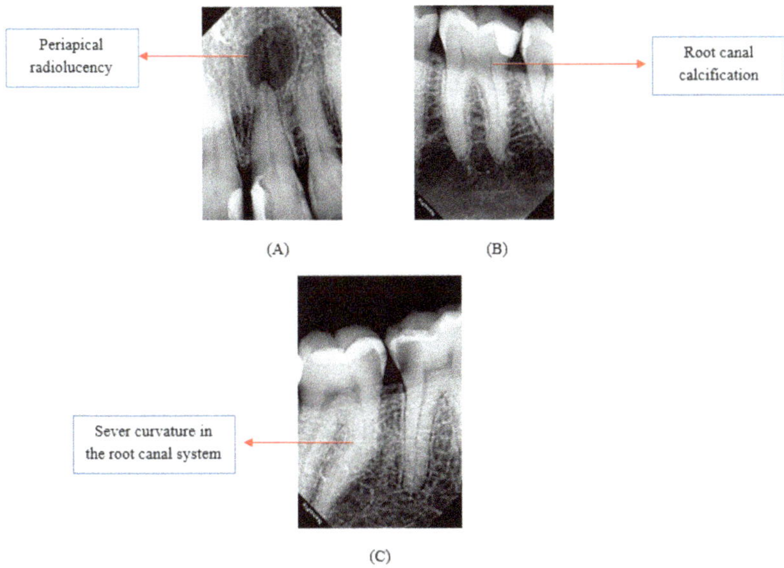

Figure 6.11. Periapical radiographs, showing (A) periapical radiolucency, (B) root canal calcification, and (C) anatomical complexity (severe curvature in the root canal system). Courtesy of the Dental Clinic Complex, College of Dentistry, King Faisal University.

This geometrical alteration can be in the range of 3.4% in periapical radiographs (Lazzerini *et al* 1996).

3. Some anatomical landmarks, such as the floor of the maxillary sinus, may overlap with some areas of the tooth being captured, such as the apex of the root (Lo Giudice *et al* 2018) (figure 6.12).

To overcome these problems, the use of cone beam computed tomography (a three-dimensional image) has recently increased; it is one of the most popular diagnostic and evaluation tools in endodontics (and will be discussed later).

The diagnosis of periodontal diseases requires radiographic images to support the clinical diagnosis. A periapical radiograph (paralleling technique) is essential for the diagnosis and treatment planning of periodontal diseases (Corbet *et al* 2009). Full-mouth periapical radiographs are recommended by the European Federation of Periodontology. Furthermore, the use of periapical radiographs allows the following to be detected regarding periodontal diseases (figure 6.13) (Tugnait *et al* 2000).

1. The bone level.
2. Furcation involvement.
3. The presence of calculus.
4. Defective restorative margin in relation to the periodontium.
5. The root morphology.
6. The root length inside the alveolar bone.
7. Evaluation of the lamina dura (e.g. widening).
8. Cemental tears.
9. The presence of root caries.

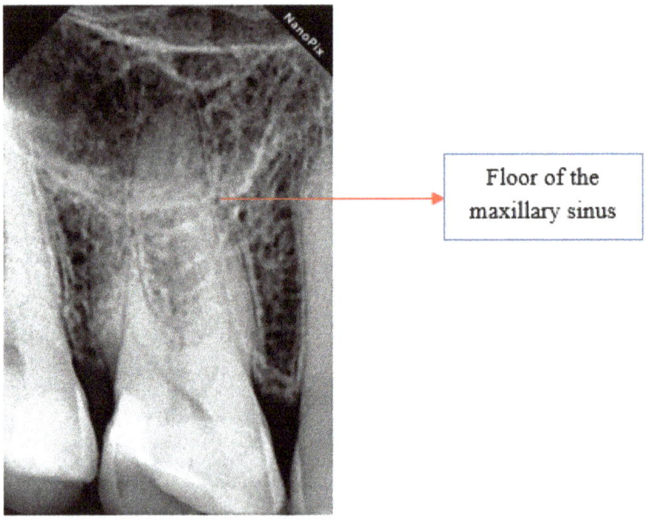

Figure 6.12. A periapical radiograph showing the maxillary first molar. The apexes of the mesiobuccal and distobuccal roots overlap the floor of the maxillary sinus. Courtesy of the Dental Clinic Complex, College of Dentistry, King Faisal University.

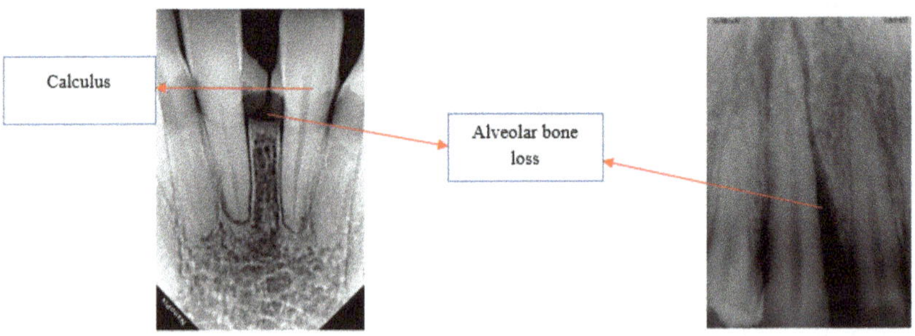

Figure 6.13. A periapical radiograph showing the presence of calculus and alveolar bone loss, indicating periodontal diseases. Courtesy of the Dental Clinic Complex, College of Dentistry, King Faisal University.

6.7.2 Bitewing radiography

The occupied space between two teeth is known as the interproximal area. The detection of any dental hard-tissue disease such as proximal dental caries or interproximal alveolar bone resorption in this area is challenging for most dentists due to the difficulty of visualizing such areas. The use of intraoral radiography, especially the bitewing radiograph, may help in the detection of such diseases.

Bitewing radiographs are intraoral radiographs that capture the crowns of the maxillary and mandibular teeth with the interproximal bone in one image (figure 6.14). The principle of a bitewing radiograph is based on placing the x-ray receptor parallel to the crowns of the maxillary and mandibular teeth and stabilizing it in place by asking the patient to bite on a bitewing beam alignment device

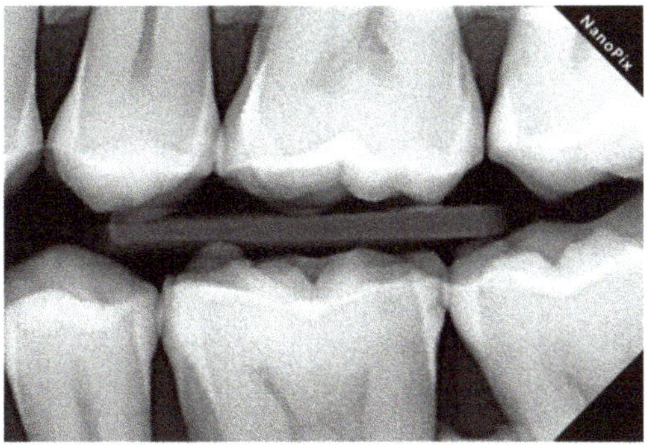

Figure 6.14. A bitewing intraoral radiograph. Courtesy of the Dental Clinic Complex, College of Dentistry, King Faisal University.

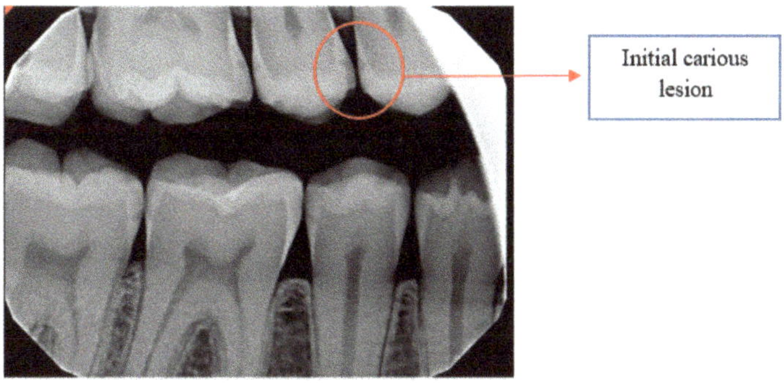

Figure 6.15. A bitewing radiograph showing an initial proximal lesion. Courtesy of the Dental Clinic Complex, College of Dentistry, King Faisal University.

(holder). The use of this holder allows the x-ray beam to run through the contact area of the teeth with ten degrees of vertical angulation of the x-ray beam. This angulation compensates for the slight angulation of the x-ray receptor opposite to the maxillary teeth (Iannucci and Howerton 2022).

Proximal carious lesions are one of the most difficult carious lesion sites to detect, especially in their initial stages (before cavitation occurs) (Luiz Mialhe *et al* 2004). Furthermore, the presence of anatomical overlaps (e.g. the presence of anatomical curvature of both crowns) may mask the presence of a carious lesion in the x-ray images (Pitts 1996). The use of a bitewing radiograph has been shown to increase the possibility of early detection of proximal carious lesions (Newman *et al* 2009) (figure 6.15). Kamburoğlu *et al* (2012) compared the efficacy of bitewing radiographs and extraoral panoramic radiographs in the detection of proximal caries. They concluded that bitewing radiographs show a superior ability to capture proximal carious lesions.

The use of a bitewing radiograph as a diagnostic tool for periodontal diseases allows better visualization of the interproximal area compared to a periapical radiograph or an extraoral radiograph such as a panoramic radiograph (Manja and

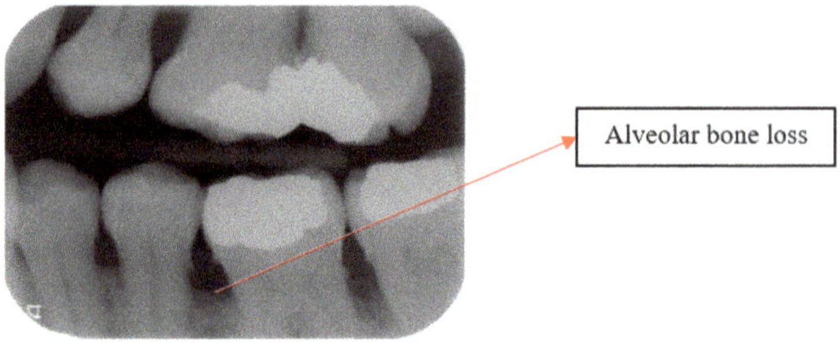

Figure 6.16. A bitewing radiograph showing crestal bone resorption between the upper and lower molars. Courtesy of the Dental Clinic Complex, College of Dentistry, King Faisal University.

Fransiari 2018). Furthermore, a bitewing radiograph allows better visualization of furcation involvement (which appears as a radiolucent area between the roots of multirooted teeth), vertical bone loss caused by trauma from occlusion, the presence of crestal bone loss due to osteoclastic activity produced by periodontal pathogens, and the presence or absence of subgingival calculus (figure 6.16) (Fiorellini *et al* 2021, Korostoff *et al* 2016). One of the drawbacks of bitewing radiography as a diagnostic tool for periodontal disease is related to its difficulty in detecting the extension of crestal bone destruction (buccal and lingual bone) as a result of the two-dimensional nature of the bitewing radiograph view compared to a three-dimensional object; hence a 3D image (cone beam computed tomography) is required (Cetmili *et al* 2019).

6.7.3 Panoramic radiography

Panoramic radiography was developed in the last century in an attempt to provide a radiograph that captures the complex maxillofacial region in one image (the entire dentition with the upper and lower alveolar jaw). The first panoramic radiograph was patented by Frank (1922), who used a narrow x-ray beam to scan the upper and lower jaw. Further improvement in the techniques and apparatus continued until 1960, when the first panoramic x-ray machine was produced (Orthopantomograph®) by Palomex (Hallikainen 1996).

A panoramic radiograph is one of the extraoral radiographs that uses extraoral receptors. It can be used as a preliminary radiographic diagnostic tool during the initial dental examination process, as it provides a primary detection of dental hard-tissue diseases such as dental caries and periodontal diseases as well as the presence of any osseous pathology (Kweon *et al* 2018, Valachovic *et al* 1986).

The sensitivity of panoramic radiography in capturing the details of anatomical features is lower compared to those of other intraoral radiographs such as periapical and bitewing radiographs (Rushton and Horner 1996). This results from the following factors (figure 6.17):

1. The superimposition of soft tissue
2. The presence of ghost shadows (shadows from soft tissues and the surrounding air)

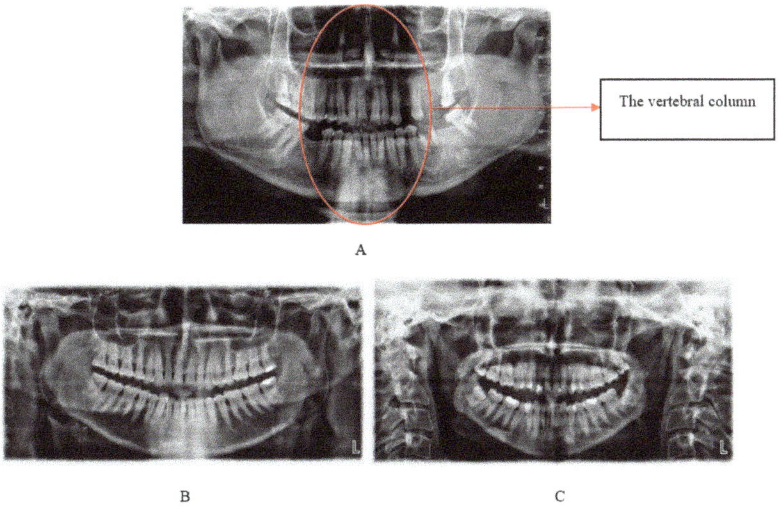

Figure 6.17. A dental panoramic view showing (A) the anterior teeth superimposed on the vertebral column, (B) and (C) dimensional changes due to patient position during x-ray exposure. Courtesy of the Dental Clinic Complex, College of Dentistry, King Faisal University.

3. Non-standardized magnification (10%–30%).
4. The superimposition of hard tissues
5. The position of the patient affects the degree of magnification.

The sensitivity of panoramic radiographs in the detection of dental caries is limited as a result of the superimposition of the hard dental tissue. Furthermore, panoramic radiographs have shown various caries detection sensitivities in different regions of the dental hard tissue; for instance, a panoramic radiograph can detect 30% of caries in the posterior (molar) region compared to only 8% in the premolar region. In addition, it shows very low sensitivity in the detection of carious lesions in the anterior region due to the superimposition of the vertebral column (Rushton and Horner 1996).

As a result of its poor ability to capture fine details, the diagnosis of endodontic diseases using panoramic radiography can be inferior to the diagnoses made using other radiographs such as periapical radiographs and cone beam computed tomography (Setzer and Lee 2021). However, panoramic radiography can be used to capture the following:

1. The presence of root or alveolar bone fractures.
2. The detection of large periapical lesions (figure 6.18).

Panoramic radiographs play an essential role as a diagnostic tool for periodontal diseases, as they can be used to assess the level of crestal alveolar bone and detect the level and extension of alveolar bone loss (figure 6.19) (Machado *et al* 2020). Some studies have found that panoramic radiography shows similar diagnostic results to those of clinical examinations (Krois *et al* 2019). Furthermore, the diagnostic value

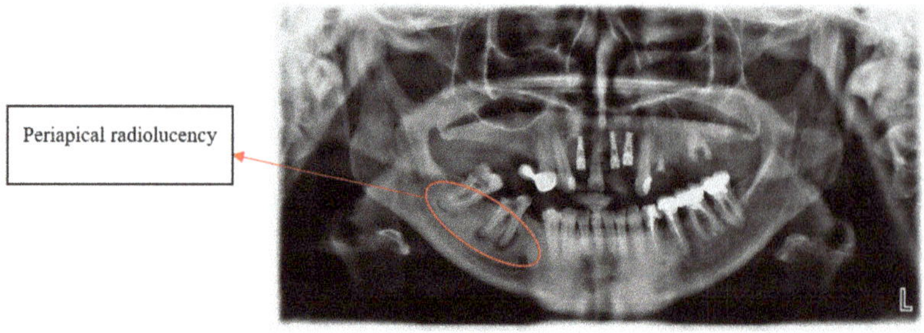

Figure 6.18. A panoramic radiograph showing periapical radiolucency at the apexes of lower right first and third molars, indicating periapical pathology. Courtesy of the Dental Clinic Complex, College of Dentistry, King Faisal University.

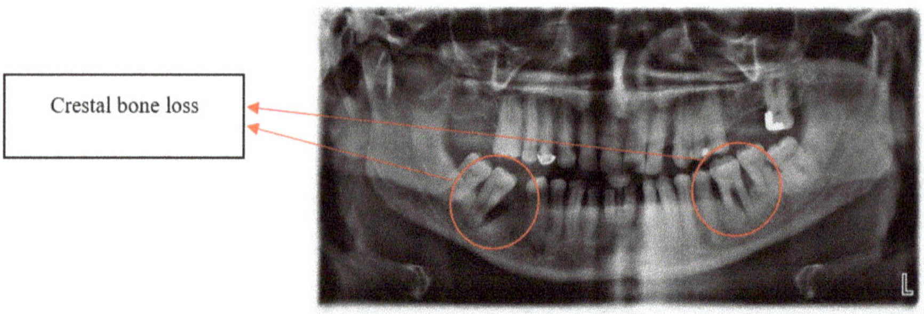

Figure 6.19. A panoramic radiograph showing alveolar (crestal) bone loss around the lower right second molar and lower left first molar, indicating periodontal diseases. Courtesy of the Dental Clinic Complex, College of Dentistry, King Faisal University.

of panoramic radiographs has been found to be similar to that of periapical radiographs in terms of the detection of radiographic features of periodontal diseases such as bone level, the presence of furcation involvement, root morphology, the presence of calculus, and the root length embedded in the alveolar bone. The periodontal ligament space can also be obtained from panoramic radiographs (Tugnait and Carmichael 2005, Tugnait *et al* 2000).

6.8 Digital radiography

In recent decades, conventional intraoral and extraoral radiographs captured in x-ray films have been used as diagnostic tools for dental hard-tissue diseases. However, one of the main drawbacks of conventional radiographs is related to the processing technique used to produce the x-ray images. The image processing technique used for conventional radiographs prevents any alteration, adjustment, or correction of any procedural errors that occur during x-ray exposure, such as overexposure or underexposure (Yoon *et al* 2018).

To overcome the drawbacks of conventional radiographs and as a result of advances in digital technology, digital radiography (digital imaging) was introduced

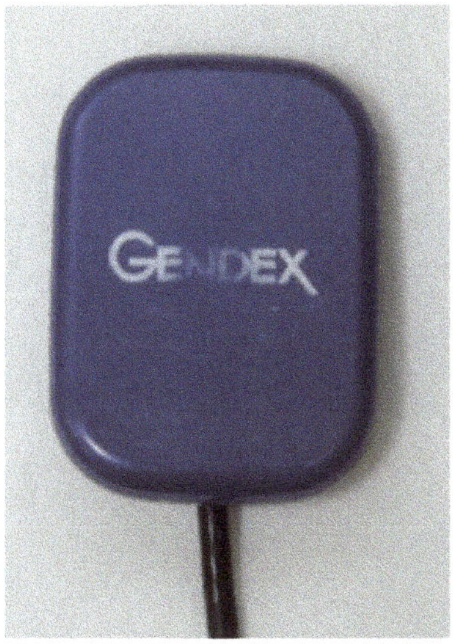

Figure 6.20. A digital (solid) x-ray receptor.

in 1984 by Dr Frances Mouyens (Parks and Williamson 2002). Since then, the concept of processing x-rays digitally has gained ground rapidly, and digital processing has now started to replace the use of conventional radiographs.

The digital processing of x-ray images (digital radiography or digital imaging) results from absorption of the x-ray photons by a solid receptor (figure 6.20). The solid receptor consists of several detectors that correspond to several pixels (similar in number) ranging between 15 and 40 microns. Furthermore, the solid receptor consist of several layers namely; X-ray scintillator layer, fiber-optic face plate, complementary metal-oxide semiconductor layer, and electronic substrate layer.

During x-ray production, the generated photons produced by the x-ray device are absorbed by the scintillator layer of the solid receptor and converted into visible light photons that are transmitted to a visible light manager (a complementary metal oxide semiconductor) layer. Within the complementary metal oxide semiconductor layer, an electrical charge is produced within each pixel by the visible light photon that was generated by the scintillator layer. The electrical charge is then converted into a voltage that corresponds to the number of photons intercepted by the pixel. Finally, the voltage in each pixel is converted into digital data that is made visible in a computer system for further processing and display (Yoon *et al* 2018).

Increasing the x-ray exposure dose results in a higher voltage output from the pixels, which then exceeds the upper voltage limit required for the digitalization of the x-ray image. Clinically, this can appear as high density in the x-ray image. However, low exposure result in reduced resolution for digitalization and hence alters the brightness of the captured x-ray image (posterization). Clinicians should use the recommended dose to prevent the disruption caused by analog-to-digital conversion errors (Yoon *et al* 2018).

Digital processing of x-ray images allows the following features to be altered or corrected, which may also be advantageous compared to conventional imaging (Wenzel 1998):

1. Brightness and contrast adjustment.
2. Data calibration.
3. Image filters.
4. Image reconstruction.
5. Geometrical errors.
6. Low radiation dose (5%–50% lower than that of a conventional radiograph).

In addition, it uses a low radiation dose (5%–50% lower than that of a conventional radiograph). Different types of dental digital radiographic images are available, such as:

Intraoral radiographs
- (i) Periapical radiographs
- (ii) Bitewing radiographs

Extraoral radiograph
- (i) Panoramic radiographs
- (ii) Lateral cephalometric radiographs

Several studies have compared the diagnostic value of digital radiography to that of conventional radiography in the detection of carious lesions. Nuvvula *et al* (2016) reviewed the literature between 1996 and 2014 and concluded that there are no conclusive results regarding the diagnostic efficacy of digital radiography compared to that of conventional radiography as a diagnostic tool to detect proximal carious lesions. Similarly, Anbiaee *et al* (2010) showed that there is no statistical difference between digital radiography and conventional radiography regarding caries detection in different sites in the tooth structure. Similar results were also obtained by Abesi *et al* (2012) and Dehghani *et al* (2017).

However, digital panoramic radiography showed superior diagnostic efficacy for periodontal diseases compared to conventional panoramic radiography. This results from the ability of the viewer to manipulate the images either by changing their brightness or contrast or by zooming, for example. Such manipulation allows better detection of any bony defect, calculus, or defects in the root morphology (Corbet *et al* 2009). Furthermore, the use of digital panoramic radiography printed on glossy paper allows five times more periapical lesions to be detected than conventional periapical radiographs (Ridao-Sacie *et al* 2007).

In conclusion, although controversy is present in the literature regarding the diagnostic efficacy of digital radiography compared to conventional radiography in detecting hard dental tissue diseases, the advantages of digital radiography are superior to those of conventional radiography.

6.9 Cone beam computed tomography

The development of computed tomography in 1973 enabled some diseases to be diagnosed or captured in a three-dimensional (3D) view (Hounsfield 1973). The advanced development of computed tomography machines has resulted in a more compact design that facilitates their use as diagnostic tools in the dental field. In 1997, Arai *et al* developed the first prototype limited cone beam computed tomography (CBCT) to be used in a dental cone beam computed tomography machine (figure 6.21) that aids in the diagnosis of different types of dental hard-tissue diseases such as periapical lesions, the locations of impacted teeth, and the evaluation of maxillary or mandibular lesions (Arai *et al* 1999). Furthermore, in 2000, a limited CBCT device was developed by Morita Co. Ltd. They created a 3D multi-image micro-CT machine that provided a 3D view of the head and neck area (Arai *et al* 2000). Around the same time, in 1998, the NewTom QR 9000 was developed to capture the maxillofacial region three-dimensionally. It worked by capturing a single scan through the use of a reciprocating x-ray that rotated around the head in 360° (Mozzo *et al* 1998).

The basic principle of CBCT image production is that an x-ray is produced in a large cone (a large volume) that extends to the whole head and neck surface while rotating only once (180°) to produce a two-dimensional image in all planes using a two-dimensional plane detector (acquisition stage). The captured image is further digitally reconstructed into a 3D image (at the reconstruction stage) to enable it to be

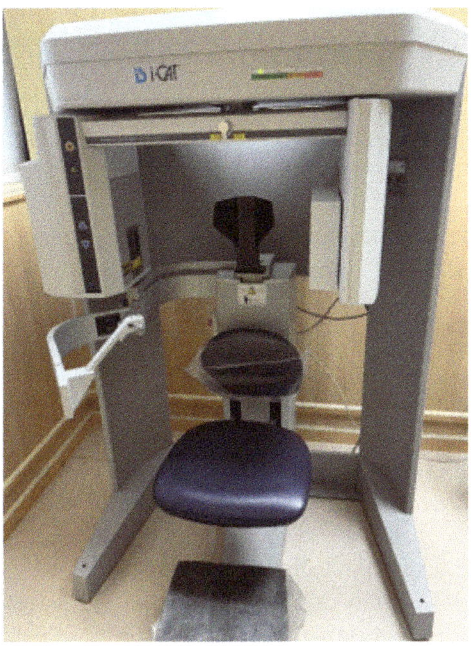

Figure 6.21. A dental cone beam computed tomography machine (I-CAT 17–19) manufactured by Imaging Sciences International LLC.

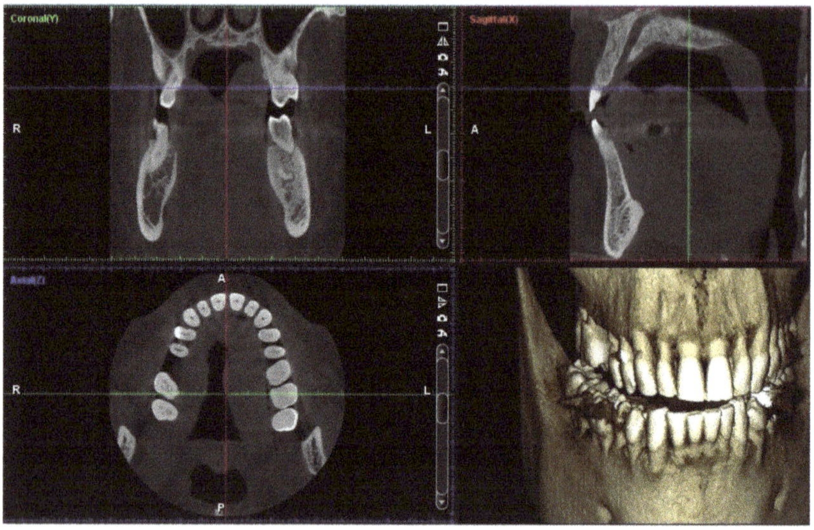

Figure 6.22. A CBCT image showing a three-dimensional image and coronal, sagittal, and axial views of a maxillofacial region. Courtesy of the Dental Clinic Complex, College of Dentistry, King Faisal University.

viewed in a three-dimensional view and three planes, namely the coronal, sagittal, and axial planes (figure 6.22) (Scarfe and Farman 2008).

The advantages of using CBCT images as a diagnostic tool for the diagnosis of oral diseases can be summarized as follows:

1. Its ability to reduce metallic artifacts
2. The patient can be in a seated position compared to to the lying position used for CT scans
3. A lower radiation dose than that of a CT scan
4. The mandible and maxilla can be captured at the same time
5. Cheaper compared to traditional computed tomography (CT scan)
6. Better resolution than that of a CT scan
7. Easy to operate and no need for a cooling room compared to CT scan.
8. No need for a cooling room.

The reduction of radiographic artifacts (metallic artifacts), such as the presence of metallic restorations or root canal filling materials, is a very important CBCT parameter for the accurate diagnosis of oral hard-tissue diseases. The presence of radiographic artifacts may significantly reduce the contrast between two adjacent objects and thus affect the quality of the CBCT image captured. Different techniques can be adopted to reduce artifacts, including:

1. *The use of an adaptive scanning technique:*

   the adaptive scanning technique allows the use of a low-voltage CBCT machine (80 kV), which can reduce metallic artifacts (Schulze *et al* 2010). Furthermore, a reduction of the voxel size or the field of view can enhance the contrast between different tissues and enhance the resolution of the captured image (Pauwels *et al* 2013).

2. *The use of a specific reconstruction algorithm:*
   specific mathematical algorithms can be used to process the raw data to analyze areas of photon starvation artifacts and beam hardening; thereby, a reconstructed image without metallic artifacts can be produced (Patel *et al* 2019).
3. *Postprocessing technique:*
   In this technique, mathematical algorithms are used to remove metallic artifacts from the captured CBCT image. However, in this case, the algorithmic processing affects a segment of the image and not the raw data. This is followed by the reconstruction of the altered segment into a new CBCT image (Parsa *et al* 2014).

Today, CBCT is used widely used as a diagnostic tool in different disciplines of dental practice, such as in treatment planning for implant placement, orthodontics, endodontics, periodontics, surgical planning, and the detection of bone pathologies.

Certain CBCT systems, such as the Accuitomo CBCT, have shown higher sensitivity in caries detection than intraoral radiographs and other types of CBCT, such as the NewTom 3G CBCT (Haiter-Neto *et al* 2008). Furthermore, the use of CBCT allows better visualization of carious lesions in a 3D view, hence minimizing the risk that undetected hidden caries fail to be visualized as a result of anatomical structural overlaps (Walsh *et al* 2021). However, its use to diagnose dental caries is limited due to its high radiation dose compared to those of other radiographs such as periapical radiographs (Kadesjö *et al* 2018).

In endodontics, unlike intraoral radiographs (digital or conventional), CBCT allows a better understanding and visualization of the internal tooth anatomy (root canal system), periapical lesions, and any bone defects in a 3D view. Some of the main advantages of using CBCT as a diagnostic tool in endodontics are its ability to detect missing canals, to identify the number of root canals and root canal orifices (root canal configuration), to identify the presence of root canal calcification (root canal obliteration)—either total or partial, to detect any bony defects such as fenestration or dehiscence, and to detect any lateral canals (figure 6.23) (Nasseh and Al-Rawi 2018, Todd 2014).

For periodontal diseases, CBCT allows better 3D visualization of the periodontal ligament space, alveolar bone defects (figure 6.24), furcation involvement, and the locations of vital anatomical structures such as the inferior alveolar canal and floor of the maxillary sinus; this leads to better diagnosis of periodontal diseases and planning for implant placement (Murali and Bhandary 2022). When the accuracy of CBCT in the detection of periodontal bone defects was compared to that of conventional radiographs, CBCT showed more accurate and precise detection of periodontal bony defects (Mark *et al* 2021).

6.10 Conclusions

Dental radiography has developed rapidly since its discovery in 1895. The dramatic advances in dental radiography have involved different aspects such as techniques,

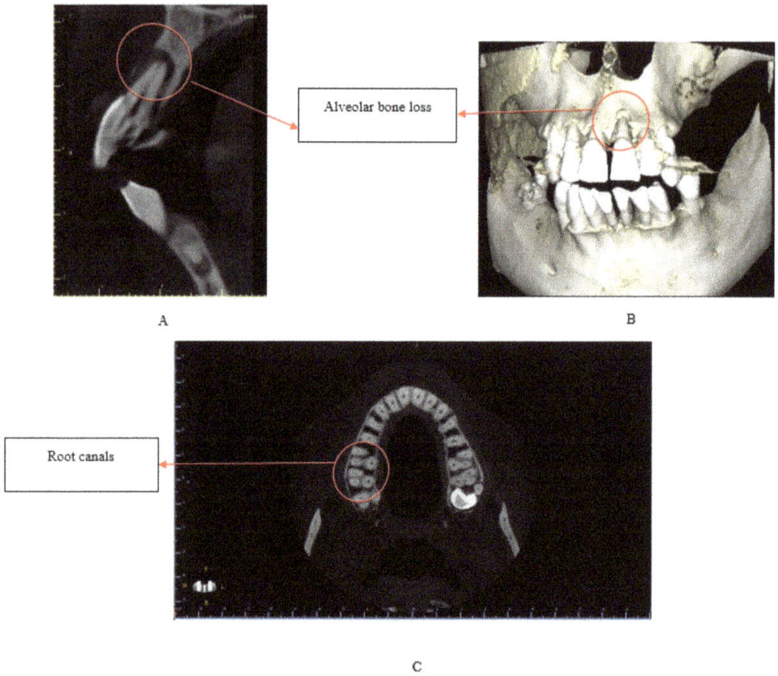

Figure 6.23. A CBCT image showing periapical radiolucency in the central left incisors in (A) sagittal plan and (B) a 3D image. (C) The number of root canals in a maxillary molar in an axial plan view. Courtesy of the Dental Clinic Complex, College of Dentistry, King Faisal University.

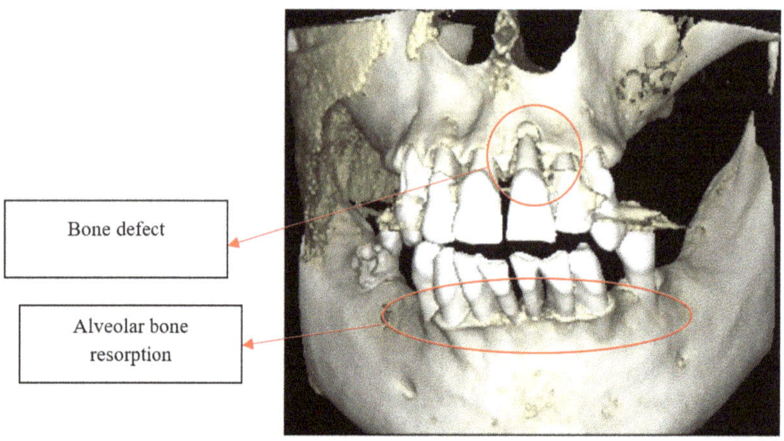

Figure 6.24. A CBCT image showing alveolar bone resorption around the lower anterior teeth and a bone defect (resorption) around the upper left central incisor. Courtesy of the Dental Clinic Complex, College of Dentistry, King Faisal University.

machines, radiation physics, and processing techniques. Furthermore, the latest developments enable dentists to diagnose and visualize dental hard-tissue diseases in a 3D view, leading to better and more accurate diagnoses. However, further enhancement is needed to meet the diagnostic requirements of dental hard-tissue diseases using simplified equipment and techniques.

References

Aas J A, Paster B J, Stokes L N, Olsen I and Dewhirst F E 2005 Defining the normal bacterial flora of the oral cavity *J. Clin. Microbiol.* **43** 5721–32

Abesi F, Mirshekar A, Moudi E, Seyedmajidi M, Haghanifar S, Haghighat N and Bijani A 2012 Diagnostic accuracy of digital and conventional radiography in the detection of non-cavitated approximal dental caries *Iranian J. Radiology* **9** 17

Abogazalah N and Ando M 2017 Alternative methods to visual and radiographic examinations for approximal caries detection *J. Oral Sci.* **59** 315–22

Anbiaee N, Mohassel A R, Imanimoghaddam M and Moazzami S M 2010 A comparison of the accuracy of digital and conventional radiography in the diagnosis of recurrent caries *J. Contemp. Dent. Pract.* **11** E025–32

Arai Y, Hashimoto K, Iwai K and Shinoda K 2000 Fundamental efficiency of limited cone-beam X-ray CT (3DX multi image micro CT) for practical use *Shika Hoshasen* **40** 145–54

Arai Y, Tammisalo E, Iwai K, Hashimoto K and Shinoda K 1999 Development of a compact computed tomographic apparatus for dental use *Dentomaxillofac. Radiol.* **28** 245–8

Berezow A B and Darveau R P 2011 Microbial shift and periodontitis *Periodontology 2000* **55** 36

Bourguignon C *et al* 2020 International Association of Dental Traumatology guidelines for the management of traumatic dental injuries: 1. Fractures and luxations *Dent. Traumatol.* **36** 314–30

Bowen W H 2013 The Stephan curve revisited *Odontology* **101** 2–8

Cetmili H, Tassoker M and Sener S 2019 Comparison of cone-beam computed tomography with bitewing radiography for detection of periodontal bone loss and assessment of effects of different voxel resolutions: an *in vitro* study *Oral Radiol.* **35** 177–83

Chan A K Y, Tamrakar M, Jiang C M, Lo E C M, Leung K C M and Chu C H 2021 A systematic review on caries status of older adults *Int. J. Environ. Res. Public Health* **18** 10662

Chen X, Daliri E B-M, Kim N, Kim J-R, Yoo D and Oh D-H 2020 Microbial etiology and prevention of dental caries: exploiting natural products to inhibit cariogenic biofilms *Pathogens* **9** 569

Corbet E, Ho D and Lai S 2009 Radiographs in periodontal disease diagnosis and management *Aust. Dent. J.* **54** S27–43

Dayo A F, Wolff M S, Syed A Z and Mupparapu M 2021 Radiology of dental caries *Dent. Clin.* **65** 427–45

Dehghani M, Barzegari R, Tabatabai H and Ghanea S 2017 Diagnostic value of conventional and digital radiography for detection of cavitated and non-cavitated proximal caries *J. Dent. (Tehran)* **14** 21

Dove S B 2001 Radiographic diagnosis of dental caries *J. Dent. Educ.* **65** 985–90

Eidt G, Waltermann E D M, Hilgert J B and Arthur R A 2020 Candida and dental caries in children, adolescents and adults: a systematic review and meta-analysis *Arch. Oral Biol.* **119** 104876

Featherstone J D 2008 Dental caries: a dynamic disease process *Aust. Dent. J.* **53** 286–91

Fiorellini J P, Sourvanos D, Sarimento H, Karimbux N and Luan K W 2021 Periodontal and implant radiology *Dent. Clin.* **65** 447–73

Frank Z A 1922 Panoramic x-ray apparatus *City: Google Patents*

Gupta A, Devi P, Srivastava R and Jyoti B 2014 Intra oral periapical radiography-basics yet intrigue: a review *Bangladesh J. Dent. Res. Educ.* **4** 83–7

Haiter-Neto F, Wenzel A and Gotfredsen E 2008 Diagnostic accuracy of cone beam computed tomography scans compared with intraoral image modalities for detection of caries lesions *Dentomaxillofac. Radiol.* **37** 18–22

Hallikainen D 1996 History of panoramic radiography *Acta Radiol.* **37** 441–5

Hardie J 1992 Oral microbiology: current concepts in the microbiology of dental caries and periodontal disease *Br. Dent. J.* **172** 271–8

Hounsfield G N 1973 Computerized transverse axial scanning (tomography): part 1. Description of system *Brit. J. Radiol.* **46** 1016–22

Iannucci J and Howerton L J 2021 *Dental Radiography-E-Book: Principles and Techniques* (Amsterdam: Elsevier Health Sciences)

Iannucci J M and Howerton L J 2022 *Dental Radiography: Principles and Techniques* (St. Louis, MO: Elsevier)

Kadesjö N, Lynds R, Nilsson M and Shi X-Q 2018 Radiation dose from X-ray examinations of impacted canines: cone beam CT vs two-dimensional imaging *Dentomaxillofac. Radiol.* **47** 20170305

Kamburoğlu K, Kolsuz E, Murat S, Yüksel S and Özen T 2012 Proximal caries detection accuracy using intraoral bitewing radiography, extraoral bitewing radiography and panoramic radiography *Dentomaxillofac. Radiol.* **41** 450–9

Kazeminia M, Abdi A, Shohaimi S, Jalali R, Vaisi-Raygani A, Salari N and Mohammadi M 2020 Dental caries in primary and permanent teeth in childrens worldwide, 1995 to 2019: a systematic review and meta-analysis *Head Face Med.* **16** 1–21

Korostoff J, Aratsu A, Kasten B and Mupparapu M 2016 Radiologic assessment of the periodontal patient *Dent. Clin.* **60** 91–104

Krois J, Ekert T, Meinhold L, Golla T, Kharbot B, Wittemeier A, Dörfer C and Schwendicke F 2019 Deep learning for the radiographic detection of periodontal bone loss *Sci. Rep.* **9** 1–6

Kweon H H-I, Lee J-H, Youk T-m, Lee B-A and Kim Y-T 2018 Panoramic radiography can be an effective diagnostic tool adjunctive to oral examinations in the national health checkup program *J. Periodontal Implant Sci.* **48** 317–25

Langland O E and Langlais R P 1995 Early pioneers of oral and maxillofacial radiology *Oral Surg. Oral Med. Oral Pathol. Oral Radiol. Endodontol.* **80** 496–511

Lazzerini F, Minorati D, Nessi R, Gagliani M and Uslenghi C 1996 The measurement parameters in dental radiography: a comparison between traditional and digital technics *Radiol. Med.* **91** 364–9

Lo Giudice R, Nicita F, Puleio F, Alibrandi A, Cervino G, Lizio A and Pantaleo G 2018 Accuracy of periapical radiography and CBCT in endodontic evaluation *Int. J. Dent.* **2018** 2514243

Luiz Mialhe F, Carlos Pereira A, Pardi V and de Castro Meneghim M 2004 Comparison of three methods for detection of carious lesions in proximal surfaces versus direct visual examination after tooth separation *J. Clin. Pediatr. Dent.* **28** 59–62

Machado V, Proença L, Morgado M, Mendes J J and Botelho J 2020 Accuracy of panoramic radiograph for diagnosing periodontitis comparing to clinical examination *J. Clin. Med.* **9** 2313

Machiulskiene V, Campus G, Carvalho J C, Dige I, Ekstrand K R, Jablonski-Momeni A, Maltz M, Manton D J, Martignon S and Martinez-Mier E A 2020 Terminology of dental caries and

dental caries management: consensus report of a workshop organized by ORCA and Cariology Research Group of IADR *Caries Res.* **54** 7–14
Manja C D and Fransiari M E 2018 A comparative assessment of alveolar bone loss using bitewing, periapical, and panoramic radiography *Bali Med. J.* **7** 636–8
Mark R, Mohan R, Gundappa M, Balaji M S, Vijay V and Umayal M 2021 Comparative evaluation of periodontal osseous defects using direct digital radiography and cone-beam computed tomography *J. Pharm. Bioallied Sci.* **13** S306
McCollough C H 1997 The AAPM/RSNA physics tutorial for residents. X-ray production *Radiographics* **17** 967–84
Mozzo P, Procacci C, Tacconi A, Tinazzi Martini P and Bergamo Andreis I 1998 A new volumetric CT machine for dental imaging based on the cone-beam technique: preliminary results *Eur. Radiol.* **8** 1558–64
Murali A C and Bhandary R 2022 Cone-beam computed tomography in periodontal diagnosis and treatment planning *J. Health Allied Sci. NU* **12** 343–9
Nasseh I and Al-Rawi W 2018 Cone beam computed tomography *Dent. Clin.* **62** 361–91
Newman B, Seow W, Kazoullis S, Ford D and Holcombe T 2009 Clinical detection of caries in the primary dentition with and without bitewing radiography *Australian Dental Journal* **54** 23–30
Nuvvula S, Bhumireddy J R, Kamatham R and Mallineni S K 2016 Diagnostic accuracy of direct digital radiography and conventional radiography for proximal caries detection in primary teeth: a systematic review *J. Indian Soc. Pedod. Prev. Dent.* **34** 300
Parks E T and Williamson G F 2002 Digital radiography: an overview *J. Contemp. Dent. Pract.* **3** 23–39
Parsa A, Ibrahim N, Hassan B, Syriopoulos K and Van Der Stelt P 2014 Assessment of metal artefact reduction around dental titanium implants in cone beam CT *Dentomaxillofac. Radiol.* **43** 20140019
Paster B J, Olsen I, Aas J A and Dewhirst F E 2006 The breadth of bacterial diversity in the human periodontal pocket and other oral sites *Periodontology 2000* **42** 80–7
Patel S, Brown J, Pimentel T, Kelly R, Abella F and Durack C 2019 Cone beam computed tomography in endodontics—a review of the literature *Int. Endodontic Journal* **52** 1138–52
Patel S, Dawood A, Whaites E and Pitt Ford T 2009 New dimensions in endodontic imaging: part 1. Conventional and alternative radiographic systems *Int. Endodontic Journal* **42** 447–62
Pauwels R, Stamatakis H, Bosmans H, Bogaerts R, Jacobs R, Horner K, Tsiklakis K and Consortium S P 2013 Quantification of metal artifacts on cone beam computed tomography images *Clinical Oral Implants Research* **24** 94–9
Pihlstrom B L, Michalowicz B S and Johnson N W 2005 Periodontal diseases *Lancet* **366** 1809–20
Pitts N 1996 The use of bitewing radiographs in the management of dental caries: scientific and practical considerations *Dentomaxillofac. Radiol.* **25** 5–16
Prados-Privado M, García Villalón J, Martínez-Martínez C H, Ivorra C and Prados-Frutos J C 2020 Dental caries diagnosis and detection using neural networks: a systematic review *J. Clin. l Med.* **9** 3579
Ridao-Sacie C, Segura-Egea J, Fernández-Palacín A, Bullón-Fernández P and Ríos-Santos J 2007 Radiological assessment of periapical status using the periapical index: comparison of periapical radiography and digital panoramic radiography *Int. Endod. J.* **40** 433–40
Robotti N 2013 The discovery of X-ray diffraction *Rend. Lincei* **24** 7–18

Rushton V and Horner K 1996 The use of panoramic radiology in dental practice *J. Dent.* **24** 185–201

Scarfe W C and Farman A G 2008 What is cone-beam CT and how does it work? *Dent. Clin. N. Am.* **52** 707–30

Schulze R K W, Berndt D and d'Hoedt B 2010 On cone-beam computed tomography artifacts induced by titanium implants *Clin. Oral Implants Res.* **21** 100–7

Seibert J A 2004 X-ray imaging physics for nuclear medicine technologists. Part 1: basic principles of x-ray production *J. Nucl. Med. Technol.* **32** 139–47

Setzer F C and Lee S-M 2021 Radiology in endodontics *Dent. Clin.* **65** 475–86

Socransky S S 1970 Relationship of bacteria to the etiology of periodontal disease *J. Dent. Res.* **49** 203–22

Tanzer J M, Livingston J and Thompson A M 2001 The microbiology of primary dental caries in humans *J. Dent. Educ.* **65** 1028–37

Todd R 2014 Cone beam computed tomography updated technology for endodontic diagnosis *Dent. Clin.* **58** 523–43

Tugnait A and Carmichael F 2005 Use of radiographs in the diagnosis of periodontal disease *Dent. Update* **32** 536–42

Tugnait A, Clerehugh V and Hirschmann P 2000 The usefulness of radiographs in diagnosis and management of periodontal diseases: a review *J. Dent.* **28** 219–26

Valachovic R W, Douglass C W, Reiskin A B, Chauncey H H and McNeil B J 1986 The use of panoramic radiography in the evaluation of asymptomatic adult dental patients *Oral Surg. Oral Med. Oral Pathol.* **61** 289–96

Velvart P, Hecker H and Tillinger G 2001 Detection of the apical lesion and the mandibular canal in conventional radiography and computed tomography *Oral Surg. Oral Med. Oral Pathol. Oral Radiol. Endodontol.* **92** 682–8

Walsh T, Macey R, Riley P, Glenny A-M, Schwendicke F, Worthington H V, Clarkson J E, Ricketts D, Su T-L and Sengupta A 2021 Imaging modalities to inform the detection and diagnosis of early caries *Cochrane Database Syst. Rev.* CD014545

Wenzel A 1998 Digital radiography and caries diagnosis *Dentomaxillofac. Radiol.* **27** 3–11

Yoon D C, Mol A, Benn D K and Benavides E 2018 Digital radiographic image processing and analysis *Dent. Clin.* **62** 341–59

Yue G, Qiu Q, Gao B, Cheng Y, Zhang J, Shimoda H, Chang S, Lu J and Zhou O 2002 Generation of continuous and pulsed diagnostic imaging x-ray radiation using a carbon-nanotube-based field-emission cathode *Appl. Phys. Lett.* **81** 355–7

Zero D T, Zandona A F, Vail M M and Spolnik K J 2011 Dental caries and pulpal disease *Dent. Clin.* **55** 29–46

Chapter 7

Tooth infections and several approaches for their treatment

Sonali Meher[1], Kushal Yadav[1] and Monalisa Mishra

Oral health is the most crucial component of a healthy lifestyle. The oral cavity harbors a large number of bacteria which continuously interact with dietary supplements, the host, and the oral environment. Bacterial colonization occurs due to this complex dynamic interaction, resulting in the formation of oral biofilm. This biofilm is responsible for oral diseases such as periodontitis and dental caries. Oral biofilm is also responsible for the formation of dental plaque. Recently developed diagnostic techniques such as fluorescence-based optical methods are used for the quantification of biofilm. The early detection of biofilm allows dentists to take personalized measures, which reduce the risk factor considerably. Antibiotics are widely used as treatments for dental issues, both for therapeutic and prophylactic reasons. Unfortunately, in last few decades, the use of antibiotics has led to the rapid emergence of antimicrobial resistance. On the other hand, nanotechnology has gained significant attention in the field of dentistry due to its enhanced physicochemical and biological properties, its biocompatibility, and its other numerous advantages. Despite of all its merits, the use of nanoparticles is limited by their toxicity, which depends on factors such as the concentration range, type, particle size, etc. This chapter illustrates the mechanism of oral biofilm formation, the diseases caused by these biofilms, and long-term sustained treatments for these problems using antibiotics and nanoparticles.

7.1 Introduction

Teeth are the important part of the human oral cavity and are composed of parts such as enamel, dentin, pulp, cementum, and periodontal ligaments [1, 2]. The basic function of teeth is to chew the food by cutting and crushing, thereby making it easy to swallow and digest. Thus, the loss of teeth due to oral disease can reduce quality

[1] Equally contributed

doi:10.1088/978-0-7503-5316-8ch7

of life in a number of ways by affecting the patterns of eating, speaking, and laughing [3, 4]. Despite the fact that they are highly preventable in nature, oral diseases have a substantial impact on the lives of individuals, communities, and society. Oral diseases are progressive and chronic in nature. For example, dental caries or decay takes place at an early age in young children, which further persists in their adulthood and later life [5].

Human saliva contains a plethora of bacterial species which adhere to the teeth, resulting in the formation of dental biofilm, also known as dental plaque [6]. Van Leeuwenhoek was the first person to observe microorganisms using a microscope in 1683. In addition to this, he also investigated his own dental plaque biofilm; since then, the study of microorganisms has attracted research attention. In the last few decades, dental biofilms and their relationships with oral diseases have been intensively studied. Bacterial species colonize the tissue surface and are implanted with a extracellular matrix formed of polysaccharides and protein. The complex of biofilm is joined together by a matrix of excreted polymeric compounds. The development of biofilm by an organism allows it to adapt to any changes in environmental conditions by altering its genetic expression.

The formation of biofilm is a dynamic process. Most biofilms are bathed by a surrounding flowing fluid, like a moss-covered rock which has a free-flowing stream of water passing over it. Mature biofilm comprises approximately 5%–25% bacterial cells and 75%–95% glycocalyx matrix [7]. Approximately 700 species of bacteria have been detected in the human oral cavity. These species are present in the oral mucosa, periodontal pockets, teeth, and tongue. The distribution of this oral microflora is not random—most species are found at preferential sites depending on the local environment. The anaerobic environment present in the periodontal pockets allow the microbes to grow [8]. This helps the development of various diseases such as dental caries and periodontitis [9]. Dental caries result from a change in nutrient status due to excessive carbohydrates, which further helps in the growth of acidogenic bacteria such as *Streptococcus mutans* [10]. Studies have shown the presence of 10^{11} microorganisms in 1 mg of dental plaque. Several other studies have shown that a pH of 6.75–7.25, a temperature of 35/36°, and a mouth cavity rich in nutrition are suitable conditions for most microorganisms to grow and form biofilm [10]. The usage of artificial implants and medical devices has no doubt improved the quality of life in humans, but on the other hand, the formation of biofilm has caused a myriad of diseases [11]. Surface roughness is a material property that affects bacterial adhesion to the surfaces of implants and the formation of biofilm. Peri-implantitis is an inflammatory condition that affects the tissue supporting implants. The natural teeth, along with implants, dentures, and dental prostheses allow biofilms to grow. Denture wearers are at a risk of denture stomatitis due to the prevalence of *Candida albicans*, a pathogenic fungus which is known to colonize the denture material poly(methyl acrylate). Nearly 65% of people with dentures have stomatitis, a condition which results in poor dental hygiene and other systemic diseases such as diabetes [12]. Dental biofilm may also influence other parts of the body. Epidemiological studies have explained the correlation between atherosclerosis, rheumatoid arthritis, *Diabetes mellitus* and periodontitis. A buccolingual section of a human tooth and its structural components are shown in figure 7.1.

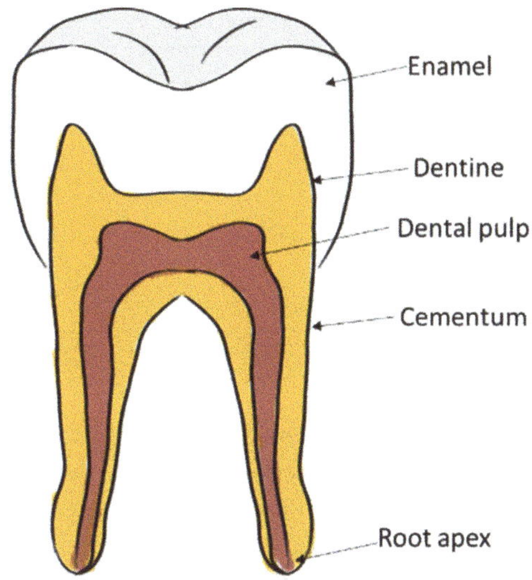

Figure 7.1. A buccolingual section of a human tooth.

7.2 Dental caries

Dental caries is the most common childhood disease and the major cause of tooth loss and oral pain. It is also referred to as cavities, which are caused by the demineralization of enamel and dentin by acids produced during the fermentation of carbohydrates by the bacteria present in the mouth [13]. In Canada, the UK, and the USA, dental caries are clearly known to impact the quality of life in children. Also in the USA, dental caries is usually to be a chronic disease which is nearly five times more prevalent than cases of asthama [14]. Dental caries is the localised deterioration of dental tissues, which are caused by the demineralisation of enamel and dentin by the acids produced during the fermentation of dietary carbohydrates [15]. It is the result of an imbalance in the physiological equilibrium between oral biofilms and tooth minerals. The process of demineralization appears on the hard tissues of the teeth; however, the disease is initiated much earlier in the biofilm that covers the tooth surface [16]. Dental caries is a condition which is affected by the factors such as the composition of the tooth, salivary flow, fluoride exposure, and dietary sugar intake. Dental caries can be prevented by cleaning the teeth on a regular basis [17]. In its initial stages, the disease is in its reversible phase, which can be stopped even if some parts of the enamel and dentin are spoiled provided that the infecting biofilm can be detached. Dental caries is a continuing disease which develops at a very slow rate. The microorganisms commonly involved in dental caries are listed in table 7.1. It is observed in both the crown and root of permanent and primary teeth (figure 7.1). It is also known to affect the enamel, cementum, and dentin. Dental caries can vary in its severity from a subclinical subsurface change at a molecular scale to lesions with dentin involvement. Bacteria such as *Streptococcus sobrinus* and *Lactobacillus spp* are present in the biofilm and produce organic acids which are synthesized as a result of carbohydrate fermentation [18, 19]. These acids eventually result in a drop

Table 7.1. Microorganisms implicated in different types of dental caries [23].

Type of dental caries	Microorganisms involved
Smooth enamel surface	*Streptococcus mutans*
Pits and fissures (irregularities)	*Streptococcus mutans, Lactobacillus* sp.
Root surface	*Streptococcus mutans, Actinomyces viscosus, Actinomyces naeslundii*
Dentinal caries	*Lactobacillus* sp., *Actinomyces viscosus, Actinomyces naeslundii*

in the local pH value, which further results in the demineralization of teeth. This step promotes the diffusion of calcium, phosphate, and carbonate and cavitation takes place progressively. The loss of mineral is further responsible for increased porosity and a widening of the gaps between the enamel which allows the acid to percolate into the tooth, resulting in demineralization [20]. The process of demineralization can be halted in its early phases by the uptake of minerals such as calcium, phosphate, and fluoride. The diffusion of calcium and phosphate in the tooth is catalyzed by fluoride. The newly crystallized surface is made of fluorapatite, i.e. fluoridated hydroxyapatite, which is more resilient to acid attack than the original tooth structure [21]. The progress, reversal, and stoppage of dental caries is basically dependent on the progression of demineralization and remineralization. These processes occur repeatedly per day in humans. Remineralization is a frequent process in which pH restoration in the biofilm takes place due to salivary flow, which acts as a buffer. Infants and toddlers are more prone to dental caries, which develop in the anterior tooth surface and progressively affect the maxillary and mandibular molars. The various factors which are responsible for dental caries include poor oral hygiene, the frequent consumption of food rich in carbohydrates, and oral medicines that are high in sugar content. Some other factors such as poverty, a lack of education, deprivation, and the use of poorly designed ill-fitting dentures also help in the formation of dental caries [22].

7.2.1 The diagnosis of dental caries

The early detection of dental caries has attracted significant interest in the field of dentistry [24]. Conventional methods of diagnosis often fail to detect the initial onset of enamel lesions, which then progress into more severe cavitation. These methods include visual inspection and tactile sensation [25]. Early detection reduces the cost of treatment and leads to minimally invasive treatment [26]. Visual inspection is a commonly implemented diagnostic method used by dentist where a tooth in a dry and clean condition should be examined under a light source. In this technique, white spot lesions, surface irregularities, enamel dissolution, cavitation, and other changes in tooth structure are assessed. Radiography is another important tooth examination method when caries lesions are not clinically visible [27]. Recent studies have shown that radiography is an effective detection method for proximal caries

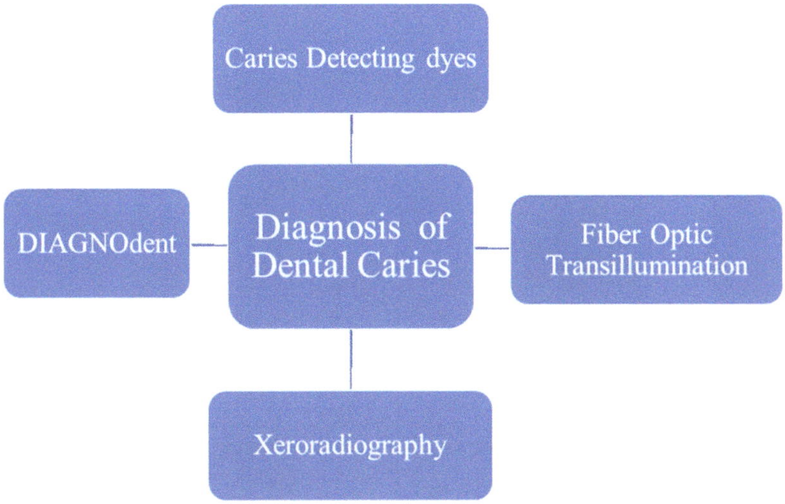

Figure 7.2. Diagnostic techniques for dental caries.

and hidden dental caries. The advance methods for early caries detection are shown in figure 7.2.

DIAGNOdent detects bacterial products using laser fluorescence technology and is essential in order to diagnose early demineralization. The fluorescent intensity is represented by numbers ranging from zero to 99. The numeric value of zero indicates the healthiest oral condition. A fiber-optic probe shines light at a wavelength of 655 nm onto the tooth surface; the light is then converted into a numeric value depending on the degree of demineralization [28]. The surface to be analyzed must be clean in order to avoid false results. DIAGNOdent can be used to detect caries with an accuracy of approximately 90%. Additionally, techniques such as wavelength-dependent fluorescence can be used for caries detection. Dental caries on hard tissue fluoresces, whereas soft tissue does not show any fluorescence. The fluorescent spectra of dentin and enamel have been measured at wavelengths of about 337, 488, 515, 613 nm. The enamel of teeth that have carious lesions exhibits a lower fluorescent intensity along with a red shift [29]. The spectral features of numerous types of caries have been detected by several researchers [29].

7.2.2 Prevention methods

1. **Oral hygiene**—The progress of dental caries can be halted by daily brushing, flossing, and rinsing, which can cut the growth of bacteria and prevent dental caries and other tooth related complications [30].
2. **Fluoride application**—The use of fluoride prevents demineralization by making the surface more resistant to acid attack. Methods of fluoride application include fluoride toothpaste, mouth rinse, and commercially available compounds such as varnishes and gels [31].
3. **Xylitol**—A high intake of sugar makes teeth more susceptible to dental caries. However, in daily life it is impossible to eliminate sugar intake from

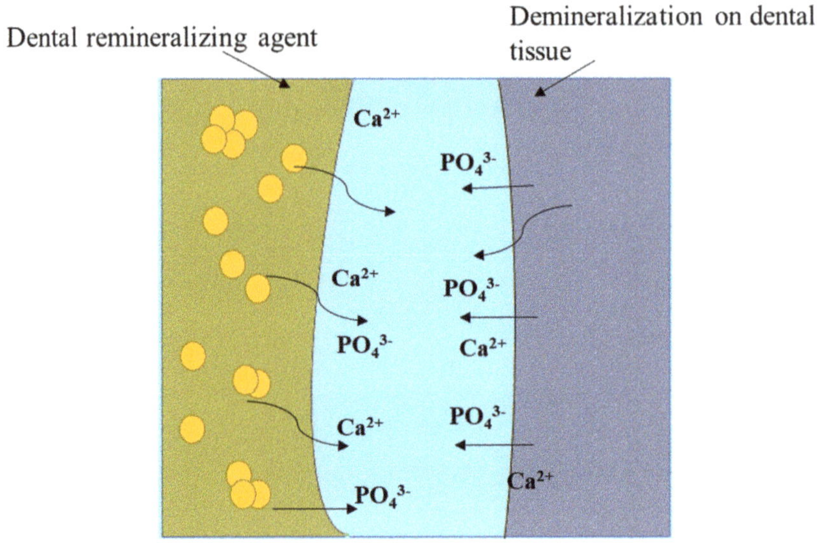

Figure 7.3. The influx and efflux of calcium and phosphate ions during remineralization and demineralization at the dental tissue surface.

our dietary consumption. Xylitol is one of the best sugar substitutes; it has a sweet flavor comparable to that of sucrose. It is non-cariogenic in nature and hence reduces the risk of caries [28].

4. **Nanocomposites**—In recent decades, nanotechnology has played a significant role in field of dentistry by improving clinical performance through the use of composite restorative materials and composite fillers. The use of silver amalgam, which is a traditional restorative material, has been limited because of its potential mercuric toxicity and other health hazards [13]. Nano silver fluoride has been used by Burns *et al* to prevent active caries in school children. Their results showed an increased efficiency in controlling dentin caries in primary teeth in comparison to a placebo. Nano zinc-based composites showed high antibacterial effects on bacteria such as *Streptococcus mutans*, although a higher concentration was used in comparison to nano silver-based fillers. Nanoparticles of monocalcium phosphate monohydrate (MCPM) and tetracalcium phosphate (TTCP) are known to release calcium and phosphate ions at the sites of caries. These nanoparticles are known for better ion release characteristics than those of their micro counterparts. Remineralizing ion release at the micro gaps between the tooth and restorative material is shown in figure 7.3.

7.3 Dental erosion

Dental erosion is damage to the hard tissues made of enamel and dentin caused by several factors, including chemical, biological, and sometimes behavioral conditions [32]. This is an irreversible condition caused by non-bacterial acids. Beverages which are acidic in nature and have other chemical properties such as low pH, mineral contents, adherence to tooth surfaces, and calcium chelation are known for their erosive potential [33]. Biological factors include the structure of the tooth, salivary flow, etc. Additional factors are dietary habits, chronic addiction to alcohol, and vigorous physical activity resulting in dehydration [34]. The sources of acid delivered to the oral system include both intrinsic and extrinsic factors [35]. Vomiting disorders such as bulimia, anorexia, and gastrointestinal disorders are common intrinsic factors. External factors for dental erosion include acidic beverages such as cold drinks, wine, fruit juices, long-term consumption of certain medicines, and the occupational environment [36]. Sweet and sour candies along with chewable vitamin C tablets make the teeth prone to erosion. Recreational drugs such as methamphetamine, ecstasy, and cocaine are also linked with dental erosion in humans. Frequent exposure of swimmers to poorly chlorinated water also creates a high risk of tooth erosion due to the low pH of the pool water [20]. In the initial stages of erosion, it may be imperceptible to detection. Frequent exposure to acid makes the process of dental erosion faster than that due to caries. Eroded teeth are characterized by the appearance of smooth glazed enamel [37]. The opening of dentinal tubules due to erosion causes severe pain, discomfort, and dentin hypersensitivity. The methods for evaluating dental erosion can be classified as:

in vitro techniques and

in vivo techniques.

In vitro techniques are methods of evaluating tooth loss due to erosion with a great deal of sensitivity, accuracy, and specificity [38]. Surface profilometry helps to quantify the surface roughness of dental tissue samples and produces two-dimensional and three-dimensional profiles of scanned surfaces. The vertical range of roughness can vary from about 300 μm to 10 mm, and this technique can detect very deep erosion pits and minor curved surfaces [39–41]. In addition, the technique of scanning acoustic microscopy uses sound waves to detect tooth abrasion, erosion, and abfraction. It uses a surface acoustic wave velocity measurement system along with a piezoelectric transducer/lens system to study the physicomechanical properties of tooth microstructures and helps in accessing mineralized tissue conditions such as dental erosion [42]. Other techniques available include iodide permeability tests, microradiography, and microdensitometric scans [43].

In vivo methods have the advantage of directly accessing dental erosion in the patient's mouth. In epidemiology, dental erosion and enamel defects can be investigated using photographs. The quality of photographs depends on the proficiency of the photographer and light reflectivity, which helps in monitoring the erosion with precision. Indices, also known as basic erosive wear examination, is another method; it comprises a scoring system in which the severity of wear is numbered using four grades ranging from zero (no surface loss) to three (more than 50% of the hard tissue lost by surface area) [44, 45].

Oral health education is an important factor in making the population aware about the complications associated with dental erosion. About 30%–50% of the population is affected by primary dentin erosion, whereas the figure ranges between 20% and 45% for permanent dentition [37, 46]. Recently, many nonrestorative approaches for the management of dental erosion have been prioritized [47]. Topical anti-erosive agents such as fluorides, calcium phosphate-based agents, and organic compounds such as poly(methyl vinyl maleic anhydride) and Carbopol are commonly used for their control of dental erosion [48]. A list of some of the commonly used topical anti-erosive agents is given in table 7.2.

Anti-erosive fluoride agents basically work by creating a protective layer around the tooth surface which is highly resistant to acid. A few of the known fluoride agents amend the salivary pellicle, thereby enhancing acid resistance. Sodium fluoride (NaF) is a monovalent fluoride which is contained at up to 1450 ppm in toothpaste [49]. A list of some of the commercially available anti-erosive agents along with the name of manufacturing company is given in table 7.3. Calcium phosphate-based agents work by providing necessary minerals which slow down the process of demineralization by making a physical barrier between the tooth and acids [50]. Calcium lactate prevents the softening of teeth by providing extra calcium ions in the saliva, which in turn reduces demineralization [51]. Organic compounds such as Carbopol [52], propylene glycol alginate [53], and palm oil [54] are derived from animals and plants or proteins such as arginine. Carbopol is an organic polymer with a negatively charged center which binds with calcium ions and forms a defensive barrier around the tooth surface.

Table 7.2. Types of topical anti-erosive agent [48].

Fluoride agents	Calcium phosphate-based agents	Organic compounds
Stannous fluoride	Calcium lactate	Carbopol
Sodium fluoride	Pyrophosphate	Palm oil
Titanium tetrafluoride	Nano-hydroxyapatite	Casein
Amine fluoride	ß-tricalcium phosphate	Arginine
Silver diamine fluoride	Linear sodium polyphosphate	Aspartame

Table 7.3. Commercially available anti-erosive agents and their manufacturers [48].

Agents	Concentration	Delivery system	Company
NaF	1100 ppm F of NaF	Toothpaste	Colgate-Palmolive Proctor & Gamble
SnF_2	1450 ppm F of NaF + SnF_2	Oral-B toothpaste	Proctor & Gamble
CHX	0.2% Chlorhexidine	Mouth rinse	Colgate-Palmolive Drogsan Pharmaceuticals

7.4 Peri-implant disease

Dental implants are becoming common these days; they combat the complications related to tooth loss [55]. Studies have shown the long-term success and stable functionalities of dental implants and their progressively increasing use in oral rehabilitation. However, the infections related to implants have also escalated due to the large numbers of people receiving dental implants [56]. This problem is also sometimes referred to as peri-implantitis, a term which was introduced almost three decades ago [57]. Dental implants are made of alloplastic materials which are incorporated for the management of tooth loss and orofacial structural loss resulting from trauma and congential defects. Osseointegrated implants and metallic implant devices made of titanium are surgically implanted in the jawbone or other regions of missing teeth [58]. These implants aim to restore the esthetic and functional characteristics of the oral cavity site [59]. These artificially introduced surfaces are prone to colonization by microbes and biofilm formation, which cause infection in the tissues supporting the implant region. The successful integration of implants has been a matter of prime importance, in which the prevention of movement is the most important criteria [60]. Loosening is the reason generally reported for the removal of implant fixtures [58]. Adell *et al* studied the success rate of implant fixtures over an observational time of five to nine years; the study included nearly 895 stable implants. Ninety-one percent of the mandibular implants remained intact. Additionally, 81% of the maxillary implants remained stable [61]. The inability of the host tissue to maintain osseointegration accounts for a significant number of implant fixture failures. Implant failures can be further categorized as early or late. The early failures are known to commence long before the osseointegration and prosthetic rehabilitation take place. The factors related to dental implant failure include fit discrepancies, premature loading, and previous failure history [62–64]. Numerous factors for implant failures are shown in figure 7.4.

The early detection of the signs and symptoms of peri-implant disease is important for its proper diagnosis and treatment [65]. Techniques such as intraoral, panoramic tomography and digital volume tomography have been demonstrated to be beneficial for radiographic interpretation [66]. The therapeutic strategies for the

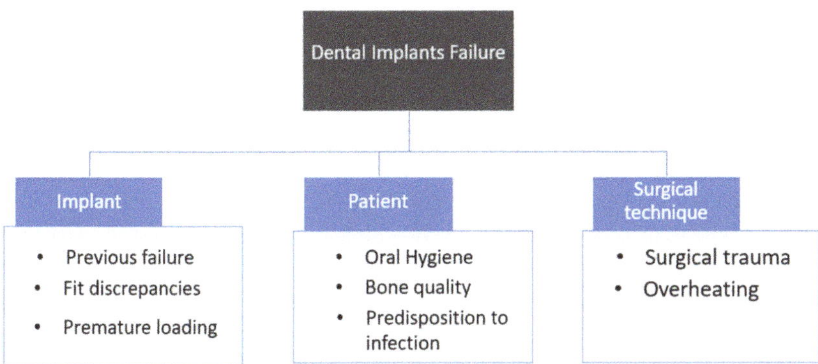

Figure 7.4 Factors for dental implant failure at an early stage.

treatment of peri-implant mucositis include plaque elimination with instruments such as carbon fiber curettes and titanium-coated curettes [67]. Mechanical debridement is another method for the removal of dental plaque and calculus that does not alter the implant surface, thereby leading to the development of a healthy mucosa [68]. The sodium carbonate air powder technique is an available method for implant surface debridement. Chlorohexidine (antiseptic) is sometimes prescribed, depending on the disease severity [69]. Antibiotics such as clindamycin, tetracycline, and ciprofloxacin are used in antibacterial therapies to decrease the numbers of pathogenic bacteria in the peri-implant pockets [70]. In recent years, there has been an increased inclination towards laser therapy for the management of peri-implant diseases. Er:YAG and CO_2 lasers have been used for such treatments [71]. Patient psychotherapy and prospects must be monitored before selecting a suitable treatment in order to obtain a fruitful outcome.

7.5 Dental abscesses

Dental abscesses are also sometimes referred to as dentoalveolar abscesses. A dental abscess is the localized accumulation of pus in the alveolar bone, which is at the root apex of a tooth. This usually takes place as a result of dental caries, failed root canal treatment, or trauma. Once microorganisms have breached the intact pulp chamber, the result is the colonization of the root canal by mixed bacteriological agents [72]. These microbes are capable of forming biofilms in the root canal, which progressively cause infection. The acute inflammation consequently leads to the formation of pus. The typical signs and symptoms of an acute dental abscess include pain, swelling, and erythema [73]. A dental abscess is a polymicrobial infection caused by *Streptococcus anginous, Anaerobic cocci, Fusobacterium*, and *Prevotella. Prevotella* are the most common isolates in significant number of studies, accounting for 10%–87% of abscesses [74]. *Prevotella nigrescens, Porphyromonas endodontalis*, and *Porhyromonas gingivalis* are some of the pathogens detected [75]. Studies have also demonstrated the presence of clostridium species such as *Clostridium hastiforme, Clostridium subterminale*, and *Clostridium histolyticum* in 2%–20% of dentoalveolar abscess [75, 76]. Certain types of new bacteria such as *Atopobium parvulum* and *Atopobium rimae*, which belong to the genus *Atopobium* have also been reported in cases of dental abcess. If not treated in their initial stages, they may spread to the potential adjacent anatomic structures and create life-threatening conditions such as a brain abscess, septicemia, sinus thrombosis, and sometimes death [72, 73, 77]. In addition, fever, intraoral and extraoral swelling, and palpitations are also observed. Delayed diagnosis due to the vagueness of the early signs and symptoms is one of the most common reasons for the high mortality rate. In the past, inappropriate sampling techniques have hampered the correct identification of the causative pathogen. The development of molecular techniques has significantly improved the routine diagnostic yield from dental abscess and has also helped to provide a good understanding of microbial bionomics [78]. Techniques such as 16S rRNA gene sequencing and DNA hybridization checkerboard techniques have improved the identification of specific microbes [75, 79]. Antibiotics such as amoxicillin, penicillin, erythromycin, and metronidazole are the most commonly prescribed medications for acute dental abscess [73]. Patients exhibiting the signs of local spread and systemic involvement should only be treated with antibiotics. Amoxicillin remains the first priority for antimicrobial treatment. Groups which are allergic to penicillin are treated with clindamycin as an alternative [80].

7.6 Periodontal diseases

Periodontal diseases are highly prevalent in the population worldwide and affect nearly 90% of the global population. Any disorder of the tissues supporting the teeth may be acquired or inherited as periodontal disease. Such disorders can be inflammatory, genetic, traumatic, or result from developmental defects [81]. Periodontal disease is mainly used to define the inflammatory conditions of gingivitis and periodontitis, which are caused by pathogens or biofilms in close proximity to the teeth [82]. Gingivitis is the trivial form of periodontal disease, which affects nearly 50%–90% of the adults globally. This condition is highly predominant and readily rescinded by adopting simple, specific oral hygiene measures. Periodontitis is the inflammation of tissues, which results in the loss of secondary connective tissues and alveolar bone. This leads to the formation of crevices and pockets between the gingiva and the tooth root [83]. In the USA, periodontitis is more prevalent among Mexican Americans than in white people. According to a survey, around 22% of the adults in the USA suffer from a mild form of periodontal infection. In addition to humans, periodontitis is also found in animals such as sheep and cattle. Dogs are among the animals most affected by this disease [84–86]. A list of organisms associated with periodontal disease is given in table 7.4.

7.7 Nanoparticles in dentistry

Nanotechnology has been one of the most active areas in the recent past due to its versatile set of applications in the field of medical science [87, 88]. Nanomaterials are particles which have at least one dimension on the order of 1–100 nm [89]. These particles possess enhanced and unique properties such as large surface-area-to-mass ratios and ultrasmall sizes, which make them suitable for antibacterial therapies [90]. They are capable of penetrating the cell walls of Gram-negative and Gram-positive bacteria, which further results in the disruption of cell functions. Other applications of nanomaterials include drug delivery, cancer therapy, biomolecule detection, and antimicrobial coatings and surfaces [91]. Nanoparticles have been gaining a lot of momentum among dental researchers because of their unique ability to withstand the harsh conditions of the oral environment [4]. Properties such as biocompatibility, a high surface area, surface chemical reactivity, and high stability have allowed the development of innovative materials with enhanced functions. Despite of all the advantages offered, some nanoparticles have limitations such as toxicity, difficulty in handling, and limited delivery [92]. The formation of cavities as a result of demineralization due to dental caries can be reversed by the application of fluoride using mouthwashes and toothpaste. The structures of nanoparticles can encapsulate or attach a required drug which can increase the level of fluoride in the oral cavities,

Table 7.4. Types of periodontal disease and their associated microorganisms [23].

Periodontal disease	Microorganism
Gingivitis	*Streptococcus sanguis* *Streptococcus milleri* *Actinomyces israelii* *Capnocytophage spp.* *Fusobacterium nucleatum*
Aggressive periodontitis	*Prevotella intermedia* *Capnocytophage spp.* *Neisseria spp.* *Aggregatibacter* *Porphyromonas gingivalis*
Adult periodontitis	*Prevotella intermedia* *Tannerella forsythia* *Fusobacterium nucleatum* *Treponema denticola* *Porphyromonas gingivalis*
Acute necrotizing ulcerative periodontitis (ANUG)	*Prevotella intermedia* *Treponema spp*

allowing remineralization. Kulshrestha *et al* used calcium fluoride nanoparticles, which are capable of inhibiting the production of exopolysaccharide by *Streptococcus mutans*. The nanoparticles used exhibited a dual effect by preventing the biofilm from further growing and also helping to remineralize tooth enamel [93]. To address the short residence time of CaF_2 nanoparticles, they can further be loaded with chitosan bio-adhesives. Ghafar *et al* incorporating CaF_2 with chitosan; the resulting material had a residence time of about 3 h during which the film remained intact. In addition, other polymers such as pectin and alginate are also used. These polymers exhibit characteristics such as biodegradability, mucoadhesion, biocompatibility, and lower toxicity [94]. Sebelemetja *et al* used other polymeric nanoparticles such as poly(ethylene glycol) and poly(lactic-co-glycolic acid) and demonstrated antibacterial and antibiofilm properties against *Streptococcus mutans* [95]. In addition to this, nanoparticles can be used as an effective approach for eradicating pathogenic bacteria and treating periodontal disease. Emmanuel *et al* used silver nanoparticles along with clarithromycin and azithromycin and reported synergistic antimicrobial efficacy against many strains of microorganisms that cause periodontal disease [96]. Nanoparticles have been used to reduce the surface contamination associated with the occurrence of peri-implantitis. Copper and silver nanoparticles possess antibacterial properties, and gold nanoparticles have been used in bone inductive adjuvants [97]. Peri-implantitis and peri-implant mucositis have also been treated using bismuth nanoparticles [98]. Titanium nanoparticles are known to prevent bacterial and fungal adhesion to implant surfaces. The success of titanium implants basically depends upon the surface characteristics, which further effect the cell adhesion, variation, and integration with tissues in their surroundings [92]. A titanium substrate in combination with chitosan and hydroxyapatite demonstrated superior antibacterial properties [99]. In addition, titanium oxide nanorod arrays which exhibited roughness, a high surface-area-to-mass ratio, and hydrophilicity showed superior antibacterial/antifungal properties. Chitosan has also been used to increase biocompatibility and bioactivity by coating the surfaces of implants [100]. It can be conjugated with substances such as collagen, hyaluronic acid, silica, hydroxyapatite, and polyacrylic acid [4]. Nanocomposites of alumina and ZrO_2 are newly available implant materials that show improved efficacy compared to ceramic materials [101]. Zirconium oxide nanoparticles can inhibit certain bacteria such as *Enterococcus faecalis (E. faecalis)* [4]. Long-term dental caries can also lead to conditions such as pulpitis and apical periodontitis. These conditions are mostly due to the bacteria and their products, which are responsible for reinfections even after root canal therapy. Microbial clean-up remains a daunting task due to the complex root canal anatomy. Silver nanoparticles showed an antimicrobial ability against *E. faecalis* [92]. The mixing of calcium silicate cement, which is a mineral trioxide aggregate, and Portland cement with silver nanoparticles enhanced the antimicrobial effect [102]. Chlorhexidine–silver nanoparticles (CHX)–AgNPs demonstrated excellent and sustained sterilization against *E. faecalis* with a bacterial inactivation rate of nearly 98.5% that lasted for more than one month [103]. Patients can significantly benefit from the recent advent of the field of nanotechnology.

7.8 Toxicity

Several studies in the past have shown that the toxicity of nanoparticles is influenced by many factors such as dosage, distribution, particle size, concentration, and duration of action [104–106]. Nanoparticles which exhibit antimicrobial properties should be delivered within a well-defined concentration range, since high concentrations of certain nanoparticles are known to have more pronounced cytotoxicity [107]. In addition to concentration, some recent studies have demonstrated that toxicity also has a strong correlation with time. Nanoparticles, due to their ultrafine size, enter the body and further accumulate in organs, resulting in the symptoms of poisoning [108]. Although a large number of studies have been conducted to explore the toxicity of nanoparticles, there is still no general agreement on limits that would standardize the toxicity of antibacterial nanoparticles [109].

7.9 Conclusions and future outlook

The book chapter aims to provide a very clear and vivid description of various oral diseases which prevail all around the globe. Nearly 3.5 billion people are affected by the chronic and progressive nature of oral diseases, which start in early childhood and linger in their later life. Diet plays an important factor in the etiology of dental caries and erosion. The development of caries is the result of organic acids available after the consumption of sugar and carbohydrates. In other inflammatory diseases such as peri-implantitis, periodontal disease, and dental abscesses, dental plaque is the major factor. Recent advancement in different diagnostic techniques have provided a remarkable delineation of tooth anatomy. Antibiotics are often the most prescribed treatments for oral infection but these may sometimes lead to resistant microbes. Some novel strategies developed in the field of nanotechnology and nanomedicine have garnered the attention of researchers, as they are very effective in controlling oral pathogens and the growth of biofilm. These smart materials have a unique ability to precisely target a specific pathogen in response to certain environmental stimuli. Auxiliary studies are needed to further evaluate the cytotoxicity and biocompatibility of these materials in humans, as the currently available data has been obtained from *in vitro* or animal studies.

References

[1] Goldberg M, Kulkarni A B, Young M and Boskey A 2011 Dentin: structure, composition and mineralization: the role of dentin ECM in dentin formation and mineralization *Front Biosci* (Elite Ed) **1** 711–35

[2] Shukla A K 2021 *Nanotechnology for Dentistry Applications* (Bristol: IOP Publishing)

[3] Lynnerup N and Klaus H D 2019 Fundamentals of human bone and dental biology *Ortner's Identification of Pathological Conditions in Human Skeletal Remains* (Amsterdam: Elsevier) 35–58

[4] Priyadarsini S, Mukherjee S and Mishra M 2018 Nanoparticles used in dentistry: a review *J. Oral Biol. Craniofac. Res.* **8** 58–67

[5] Peres M A, Macpherson D, Weyant L M, Daly R J, Venturelli B and Mathur R M R *et al* 2019 Oral diseases: a global public health challenge *Lancet* **394** 249–60

[6] Allaker R P 2010 Critical review in oral biology and medicine: the use of nanoparticles to control oral biofilm formation *J. Dent. Res.* **89** 1175–86

[7] Huang R, Li M and Gregory R L 2011 Bacterial interactions in dental biofilm *Virulence* **2** 435–44 Boca Raton, FLTaylor and Francispp

[8] Larsen T and Fiehn N-E 2017 Dental biofilm infections—an update *APMIS* **125** 376–84

[9] Lim G, Janu U, Chiou L-L, Gandhi K K, Palomo L and John V 2020 Periodontal health and systemic conditions *Dent. J.* **8** 130

[10] Haque M, Sartelli M and Haque S Z 2019 Dental infection and resistance-global health consequences *Dent. J.* **7** 22

[11] Franjić S 2021 Damage in dentistry *J. Health Care Res.* **2** 146–52

[12] Berger D, Rakhamimova A, Pollack A and Loewy Z 2018 Oral biofilms: development, control, and analysis *High-Throughput* **7** 24

[13] Chaughule R, Raorane D, Pednekar S and Dashaputra R 2018 Nanocomposites and their use in dentistry *Dental Applications of Nanotechnology* (Cham: Springer International Publishing) 59–79

[14] Pitts N B, Zero D T, Marsh P D, Ekstrand K, Weintraub J A and Ramos-Gomez F *et al* 2017 Dental caries *Nat. Rev. Dis. Primers* **3** 17031

[15] Agustsdottir H, Gudmundsdottir H, Eggertsson H, Jonsson S H, Gudlaugsson J O and Saemundsson S R *et al* 2010 Caries prevalence of permanent teeth: a national survey of children in Iceland using ICDAS *Community Dent. Oral Epidemiol.* **38** 299–309

[16] Selwitz R H 2007 Dental caries *Lancet* **369** 51–9

[17] Fejerskov O, Nyvad B and Kidd E (ed) 2015 Prologue 3 *Dental Caries: The Disease and its Clinical Management, 3rd Edition* (Hoboken, NJ: Wiley)

[18] Tinanoff N, Kanellis M J and Vargas C M 2002 Current understanding of the epidemiology, mechanisms, and prevention of dental caries in preschool children *Pediatr. Dent.* **24** 543–51

[19] Krol D M 2003 Dental caries, oral health, and pediatricians *Curr. Probl. Pediatr. Adolesc. Health Care* **33** 253–70

[20] Moynihan P and Petersen P E 2004 Diet, nutrition and the prevention of dental diseases *Public Health Nutr* **7** 201–26

[21] Ahmadian E, Shahi S, Yazdani J, Maleki Dizaj S and Sharifi S 2018 Local treatment of the dental caries using nanomaterials *Biomed. Pharmacother.* **108** 443–7

[22] Watt R G, Mathur M R, Aida J, Bönecker M, Venturelli R and Gansky S A 2018 Oral health disparities in children: a canary in the coalmine? *Pediatr. Clin. North Am.* **65** 965–79

[23] Patil S, Rao R S, Sanketh D S and Amrutha N 2013 Microbial flora in oral diseases *J. Contemp. Dent. Pract.* 14 1202–8

[24] Pretty I A and Ekstrand K R 2016 Detection and monitoring of early caries lesions: a review *Eur. Arch. Paediatr. Dent.* **17** 13–25

[25] Yılmaz H and Keleş S 2018 Recent methods for diagnosis of dental caries in dentistry *Meandros Med. Dent. J.* **19** 1–8

[26] Ismail A I, Tellez M, Pitts N B, Ekstrand K R, Ricketts D and Longbottom C *et al* 2013 Caries management pathways preserve dental tissues and promote oral health *Community Dent. Oral Epidemiol.* **41** e12–e40

[27] Marinova-Takorova M, Anastasova R and Panov V E 2014 Comparative evaluation of the effectiveness of five methods for early diagnosis of occlusal caries lesions—*in vitro* study. *J. IMAB* **20** 533–6

[28] Lee Y 2013 Diagnosis and prevention strategies for dental caries *J. Lifestyle Med.* **3** 107–9

[29] Ko C C, Yi D H, Lee D J, Kwon J, Garcia-Godoy F and Kwon Y H 2017 Diagnosis and staging of caries using spectral factors derived from the blue laser-induced autofluorescence spectrum *J. Dent.* **67** 77–83

[30] Bayrak S, Tuloglu N, Bicer H and Tuncsen E 2017 Effect of fluoride varnish containing CPP-ACP on preventing enamel erosion *Scanning* **2017** 1897825

[31] Lussi A, Buzalaf M A R, Duangthip D, Anttonen V, Ganss C and João-Souza S H *et al* 2019 The use of fluoride for the prevention of dental erosion and erosive tooth wear in children and adolescents *Eur. Arch. Paediatr. Dent.* **20** 517–27

[32] Warreth A, Abuhijleh E, Almaghribi M A, Mahwal G and Ashawish A 2020 Tooth surface loss: a review of literature *Saudi Dent. J.* **32** 53–60

[33] Okunseri C, Wong M C M, Yau D T W, McGrath C and Szabo A 2015 The relationship between consumption of beverages and tooth wear among adults in the United States *J. Public Health Dent.* **75** 274–81

[34] Sato T, Fukuzawa Y, Kawakami S, Suzuki M, Tanaka Y and Terayama H *et al* 2021 The onset of dental erosion caused by food and drinks and the preventive effect of alkaline ionized water *Nutrients* **13** 3440

[35] Kanzow P, Wegehaupt F J, Attin T and Wiegand A 2016 Etiology and pathogenesis of dental erosion *Quintessence Int.* **47** 275–8
[36] Nijakowski K, Zdrojewski J, Nowak M, Podgórski F and Surdacka A 2022 Regular physical activity and dental erosion: a systematic review *Appl. Sci.* **12** 1099
[37] Lussi A, Schlueter N, Rakhmatullina E and Ganss C 2011 Dental erosion—an overview with emphasis on chemical and histopathological aspects *Caries Res.* **45** 2–12
[38] Joshi M 2016 Techniques to Evaluate Dental Erosion: A Systematic Review of Literature *J. Clin. Diagn. Res.* **10** ZE01–7
[39] Rodriguez J M, Curtis R v and Bartlett D W 2009 Surface roughness of impression materials and dental stones scanned by non-contacting laser profilometry *Dent. Mater.* **25** 500–5
[40] Azzopardi A, Bartlett D W, Watson T F and Sherriff M 2004 The surface effects of erosion and abrasion on dentine with and without a protective layer *Br. Dent. J.* **196** 351–4
[41] Diaci J 2008 Laser profilometry for the characterization of craters produced in hard dental tissues by Er: YAG and Er, Cr: YSGG lasers *J. Laser Health Acad.* **2008** 2 https://www.laserandhealthacademy.com/en/journal/?id=957&type=1
[42] Chen Y L, Chang H H, Chiang Y C and Lin C P 2013 Application and development of ultrasonics in dentistry *J. Formos. Med. Assoc.* **112** 659–65
[43] Hafström-Björkman U *et al* 1996 Comparison of laser fluorescence and longitudinal microradiography for quantitative assessment of *in vitro* enamel caries *Caries Res.* **26** 241–7
[44] Bardsley P F 2008 The evolution of tooth wear indices *Clin. Oral Investig* **12** 15–9
[45] Mulic A, Tveit A B, Wang N J, Hove L H, Espelid I and Skaare A B 2010 Reliability of two clinical scoring systems for dental erosive wear *Caries Res.* **44** 294–9
[46] Jakubovics N S, Goodman S D, Mashburn-Warren L, Stafford G P and Cieplik F 2021 The dental plaque biofilm matrix *J. Periodontol. 2000* **86** 32–56
[47] Øilo M and Bakken V 2015 Biofilm and dental biomaterials *Materials.* **8** 2887–900
[48] Chawhuaveang D D, Yu O Y, Yin I X, Lam W Y H and Chu C H 2022 Topical agents for nonrestorative management of dental erosion: a narrative review *Healthcare (Basel)* **10** 1413
[49] Ren Y F, Liu X, Fadel N, Malmstrom H, Barnes V and Xu T 2011 Preventive effects of dentifrice containing 5000 ppm fluoride against dental erosion *in situ J. Dent.* **39** 672–8
[50] Viana Í E L, Lopes R M, Silva F R O, Lima N B, Aranha A C C and Feitosa S *et al* 2020 Novel fluoride and stannous-functionalized β-tricalcium phosphate nanoparticles for the management of dental erosion *J. Dent.* **92** 103263
[51] Turssi C P, Hara A T, Amaral F L B, França F M G and Basting R T 2014 Calcium lactate pre-rinse increased fluoride protection against enamel erosion in a randomized controlled *in situ* trial *J. Dent.* **42** 534–9
[52] Ávila D M, da S, Zanatta R F, Scaramucci T, Aoki I V, Torres C R G and Borges A B 2017 Influence of bioadhesive polymers on the protective effect of fluoride against erosion *J. Dent.* **56** 45–52
[53] Bezerra S J C, João-Souza S H, Aoki I v, Borges A B, Hara A T and Scaramucci T 2019 Anti-erosive effect of solutions containing sodium fluoride, stannous chloride, and selected film-forming polymers *Caries Res.* **53** 305–13

[54] Ionta F Q, Alencar C R B, de, Santos N M, dos, Bergantin B T P, Val P P and Honório H M *et al* 2018 Effect of palm oil alone or associated to stannous solution on enamel erosive–abrasive wear: a randomized *in situ*/*ex vivo* study *Arch. Oral Biol.* **95** 68–73

[55] Heitz-Mayfield L J A 2008 Peri-implant diseases: diagnosis and risk indicators *J. Clin. Periodontol.* **35** 292–304

[56] Ramachandran M, Sivaji C and Sriram S 2022 An overview of dental implant and its bio mineralization screening *Pharm. Sci. Res.* **1** 34–41

[57] Zohrabian V M and Abrahams J J 2015 Inflammatory diseases of the teeth and jaws *Semin. Ultrasound CT MRI* **36** 434–43

[58] Pye A D, Lockhart D E A, Dawson M P, Murray C A and Smith A J 2009 A review of dental implants and infection *J. Hosp. Infect.* **72** 104–10

[59] Fu J-H and Wang H-L 2020 Breaking the wave of peri-implantitis *Periodontol. 2000* **84** 145–60

[60] Klinge B, Klinge A, Bertl K and Stavropoulos A 2018 Peri-implant diseases *Eur. J. Oral Sci.* **126** 88–94

[61] Adell R, Lekholm U, Rockler B and Brånemark P I 1981 A 15-year study of osseointegrated implants in the treatment of the edentulous jaw *Int. J. Oral Surg.* **10** 387–416

[62] Romandini M, Lima C, Pedrinaci I, Araoz A, Soldini M C and Sanz M 2021 Prevalence and risk/protective indicators of peri-implant diseases: a university-representative cross-sectional study *Clin. Oral Implants Res.* **32** 112–22

[63] Rakic M, Galindo-Moreno P, Monje A, Radovanovic S, Wang H L and Cochran D *et al* 2018 How frequent does peri-implantitis occur? A systematic review and meta-analysis *Clin. Oral Investig.* **22** 1805–16

[64] Alassy H, Parachuru P and Wolff L 2019 Peri-implantitis diagnosis and prognosis using biomarkers in peri-implant crevicular fluid: a narrative review *Diagnostics.* **9** 214

[65] Romanos G E, Javed F, Delgado-Ruiz R A and Calvo-Guirado J L 2015 Peri-implant diseases: a review of treatment interventions *Dent. Clin. N. Am.* **59** 157–78

[66] Das D and Shenoy N 2022 Peri-implant diseases *J. Health Allied Sci. NU* **12** 223–9

[67] Thöne-Mühling M, Swierkot K, Nonnenmacher C, Mutters R, Flores-de-Jacoby L and Mengel R 2010 Comparison of two full-mouth approaches in the treatment of peri-implant mucositis: a pilot study *Clin. Oral Implants Res.* **21** 504–12

[68] Persson G R, Samuelsson E, Lindahl C and Renvert S 2010 Mechanical non-surgical treatment of peri-implantitis: a single-blinded randomized longitudinal clinical study. II. Microbiological results *J. Clin. Periodontol.* **37** 563–73

[69] Lang P and Brecx M C 1986 Chlorhexidine digiuconate—an agent for chemicai plaque control and prevention of gingival inflammation *J. Periodontal Res. Suppl.* **21** 74–89

[70] Luengo F, Solonko M, Sanz-Esporrín J, Sanz-Sánchez I, Herrera D and Sanz M 2022 Clinical, microbiological, and biochemical impact of the surgical treatment of peri-implantitis—a prospective case series *J. Clin. Med.* **11** 4699

[71] Mailoa J, Lin G H, Chan H L, MacEachern M and Wang H L 2014 Clinical outcomes of using lasers for peri-implantitis surface detoxification: a systematic review and meta-analysis *J. Periodontol.* **85** 1194–202

[72] Robertson D and Smith A J 2009 The microbiology of the acute dental abscess *J. Med. MicroBiol.* **58** 155–62

[73] Shweta 2013 Dental abscess: a microbiological review *Dent. Res. J. (Isfahan)* **10** 585–91

[74] Sherrard L J, Graham K A, McGrath S J, McIlreavey L, Hatch J and Muhlebach M S *et al* 2013 Antibiotic resistance in prevotella species isolated from patients with cystic fibrosis *J. Antimicrob. Chemother.* **68** 2369–74

[75] Böttger S, Zechel-Gran S, Schmermund D, Streckbein P, Wilbrand J-F and Knitschke M *et al* 2021 Microbiome of odontogenic abscesses *Microorganisms* **9** 1307

[76] Kuriyama T 2007 Antimicrobial susceptibility of 800 anaerobic isolates from patients with dentoalveolar infection to 13 oral antibiotics *Oral Microbiol. Immunol.* **22** 285–8

[77] Bik E M, Long C D, Armitage G C, Loomer P, Emerson J and Mongodin E F *et al* 2010 Bacterial diversity in the oral cavity of 10 healthy individuals *ISME J.* **4** 962–74

[78] Chen H and Jiang W 2014 Application of high-throughput sequencing in understanding human oral microbiome related with health and disease *Front. MicroBiol.* **5** 508

[79] Sakamoto M 2006 Molecular analysis of bacteria in asymptomatic and symptomatic endodontic infections *Oral Microbiol. Immunol.* **21** 112–22

[80] Fouad F, Rivera E M, Walton R E and Farmington C 1996 *Oral Surg. Oral Med. Oral Pathol. Oral Radiol. Endod.* **81** 590–5

[81] Armitage G C 2004 Periodontal diagnoses and classification of periodontal diseases *Periodontol 2000* **34** 9–21

[82] Ray R R 2022 Periodontitis: an oral disease with severe consequences *Appl. Biochem. Biotechnol.* **195** 17–32

[83] Listgarten M A 1988 The role of dental plaque in gingivitis and periodontitis *J. Clin. Periodontol.* **15** 485–7

[84] Chapple I L C, van der Weijden F, Doerfer C, Herrera D, Shapira L and Polak D *et al* 2015 Primary prevention of periodontitis: managing gingivitis *J. Clin. Periodontol.* **42** S71–6

[85] Larsen T and Fiehn N E 2017 Dental biofilm infections – an update *APMIS*Vol. 125 (Blackwell Munksgaard) p 376–84

[86] Shahabouee M, Rismanchian M, Yaghini J, Babashahi A, Badrian H and Goroohi H 2012 Microflora around teeth and dental implants *Dent. Res. J.* **2** 215–20

[87] Ramsden J J 2016 What is nanotechnology? *Nanotechnology* (Amsterdam: Elsevier) pp 1–18

[88] Directorate-General for Research and Innovation (European Commission) 2012 *Nanotechnologies: Principles, Applications, Implications and Hands-on Activities (A compendium for educators)* (Luxembourg: Publications Office of the European Union) https://op.europa.eu/s/yNuj

[89] Bhushan J and Maini C 2019 Nanoparticles: a promising novel adjunct for dentistry *Indian J. Dent. Sci.* **11** 167

[90] Rahimi-Iman A 2020 Advances in functional nanomaterials science *Ann. Phys.* **532** 2000015

[91] Mahanta U, Khandelwal M and Deshpande A S 2021 Antimicrobial surfaces: a review of synthetic approaches, applicability and outlook *J. Mater. Sci.* **56** 17915–41

[92] Kulshrestha S, Khan S, Hasan S, Khan M E, Misba L and Khan A U 2016 Calcium fluoride nanoparticles induced suppression of *Streptococcus mutans* biofilm: an *in vitro* and *in vivo* approach *Appl. Microbiol. Biotechnol.* **100** 1901–14

[93] Ghafar H, Khan M I, Sarwar H S, Yaqoob S, Hussain S Z and Tariq I *et al* 2020 Development and characterization of bioadhesive film embedded with lignocaine and calcium fluoride nanoparticles *AAPS PharmSciTech* **21** 60

[94] Sebelemetja M, Moeno S and Patel M 2020 Anti-acidogenic, anti-biofilm and slow release properties of *Dodonaea viscosa* var. *angustifolia* flavone stabilized polymeric nanoparticles *Arch. Oral Biol.* **109** 104586

[95] Emmanuel R, Palanisamy S, Chen S M, Chelladurai K, Padmavathy S and Saravanan M *et al* 2015 Antimicrobial efficacy of green synthesized drug blended silver nanoparticles against dental caries and periodontal disease causing microorganisms *Mater. Sci. Eng.*, C **56** 374–9

[96] Jadhav K, Rajeswari H R, Deshpande S, Jagwani S, Dhamecha D and Jalalpure S *et al* 2018 Phytosynthesis of gold nanoparticles: characterization, biocompatibility, and evaluation of its osteoinductive potential for application in implant dentistry *Mater. Sci. Eng.* C **93** 664–70

[97] Gosau M, Haupt M, Thude S, Strowitzki M, Schminke B and Buergers R 2016 Antimicrobial effect and biocompatibility of novel metallic nanocrystalline implant coatings *J. Biomed. Mater. Res.* B **104** 1571–9

[98] Moraes G, Zambom C and Siqueira W L 2021 Nanoparticles in dentistry: a comprehensive review *Pharmaceuticals* **14** 752

[99] Martinez E, Ishikawa G, de Lemos A, Barbosa Bezerra F, Sperandio M and Napimoga M 2017 Evaluation of a titanium surface treated with hydroxyapatite nanocrystals on osteoblastic cell behavior: an *in vitro* study *Int. J. Oral Maxillofac. Implants* **33** 597–602

[100] Cheng Y F, Zhang J Y, Wang Y B, Li C M, Lu Z S and Hu X F *et al* 2019 Deposition of catechol-functionalized chitosan and silver nanoparticles on biomedical titanium surfaces for antibacterial application *Mater. Sci. Eng.* C **98** 649–56

[101] Schmalz G, Hickel R, van Landuyt K L and Reichl F X 2017 Nanoparticles in dentistry *Dent. Mater.* **33** 1298–314 1298–314

[102] Nam K Y 2017 Characterization and antimicrobial efficacy of Portland cement impregnated with silver nanoparticles *J. Adv. Prosthodont.* **9** 217–23

[103] Zheng T, Huang X, Chen J, Feng D, Mei L and Huang Y *et al* 2018 A liquid crystalline precursor incorporating chlorhexidine acetate and silver nanoparticles for root canal disinfection *Biomater. Sci.* **6** 596–603

[104] Weng S, Zhao X, Liu G, Guan Y, Wu F and Luo Y 2018 Synthesis, characterization, antibacterial activity in dark and *in vitro* cytocompatibility of Ag-incorporated TiO_2 microspheres with high specific surface area *J. Mater. Sci. Mater. Med.* **29** 50

[105] Jin J, Zhang L, Shi M, Zhang Y and Wang Q 2017 Ti-GO-Ag nanocomposite: the effect of content level on the antimicrobial activity and cytotoxicity *Int. J. Nanomed.* **12** 4209–24

[106] Yang Y, Ren S, Zhang X, Yu Y, Liu C and Yang J *et al* 2018 Safety and efficacy of PLGA ($Ag–Fe_3O_4$)-coated dental implants in inhibiting bacteria adherence and osteogenic inducement under a magnetic field *Int. J. Nanomed.* **13** 3751–62

[107] Chen R, Han Z, Huang Z, Karki J, Wang C and Zhu B *et al* 2017 Antibacterial activity, cytotoxicity and mechanical behavior of nano-enhanced denture base resin with different kinds of inorganic antibacterial agents *Dent. Mater. J.* **36** 693–9

[108] Vilarrasa J, Delgado L M, Galofré M, Àlvarez G, Violant D and Manero J M *et al* 2018 *In vitro* evaluation of a multispecies oral biofilm over antibacterial coated titanium surfaces *J. Mater. Sci. Mater. Med.* **29** 164

[109] Mishra M 2021 Neurotoxicity of nanomaterials used in the field of dentistry *Nanotechnology for Dentistry Applications* (Bristol: IOP Publishing) 13

Milton Keynes UK
Ingram Content Group UK Ltd.
UKHW051503171023
430775UK00003B/10

9 780750 353144